RADIANT RELIEF

RADIANT RELIEF

A CASE FOR
A Better Solution
TO
Chronic Pain

—

P. BRENDON LUNDBERG,
WITH DAVID B. FARLEY, MD

Sollievo
Publishing LLC

RADIANT RELIEF

A Case for a Better Solution to Chronic Pain

ISBN   978-1-5445-0089-8 *Paperback*

978-1-5445-0088-1 *Ebook*

CRISTINA—

I HOPE YOU ENJOY THIS
BOOK. IT'S A GIFT. TO HELP
GROW AWARENESS AND INFLUENCE
FOR RADIANT WOULDN'T BE
POSSIBLE WITHOUT YOUR
FAMILY'S SUPPORT. LET'S
CHANGE THE WORLD, EASE
SUFFERING AND INCREASE JOY,
CONNECTION AND PRODUCTIVITY
IN THE LIVES OF MILLIONS!

— BRENDON

CONTENTS

Visit RadiantReliefBook.com to download free resources to help you better understand and manage chronic pain.

This valuable content is based on the latest scientific understanding of chronic pain.

These resources are ideal both for pain sufferers and for those who care for them, including medical professionals.

ACKNOWLEDGMENTS

———

For my wife, Rachel, because entrepreneurship is hard, especially for the spouse, especially in the years or decades it takes before it all actually comes together.

For my kids, Lauren, Julien, and Maude, I hope you'll fight for your dreams and always try to make this world a better place.

For my parents, Phil and Rae Lundberg, who taught me love, and who have always honored my independence and celebrated my individuality.

For Barb Gittus-Servino, for being the first boss that truly inspired me. I wish you were here to see this.

For Brendon Burchard and those in the High Performance Mastermind for helping me know myself and gain the clarity and courage to pursue my dreams with joy and gratitude.

For Joe Polish and the Genius Network for helping expand my thinking and giving me a network of inspiration.

INTRODUCTION

WHY YOU SHOULD READ THIS BOOK

———

Chronic pain is a complicated problem. But if you're reading this, you already know how complicated it can be, maybe because you are living with chronic pain or you care for someone who is. It is now commonplace to hear about chronic pain in media outlets, especially the devastating epidemic of opioid addiction.

I am a chronic pain sufferer myself. I have a condition of the spine which causes pain and stiffness in my low back, and which has caused intense pain to radiate down my leg and into my groin. Movement, sleep, activities, and my attitude have all been compromised because of pain. Yet my pain is mild compared to many. I see so many people who have had their lives robbed by pain—robbed of comfort, robbed of function, productivity, joy, presence, hope, and more. No one likes to be robbed. No one likes to see someone they care about be robbed of a full and thriving life.

It stirs something within us: a call to action, a need for change.

And that is why I wrote this book and have dedicated years of my life to building a better solution through Radiant Pain Relief Centres, because chronic pain is robbing too many of us of a full life, and I am on a mission to change that.

Indeed, chronic pain is complicated. Complicated in how it intervenes in our lives, complicated in its understanding and origin, and complicated in how healthcare has grown to understand and address it. Because of this, I will touch on some of these aspects related to the science of pain, to healthcare, and to business. I know that chronic pain sufferers, and those that care for them, are two things if nothing else:

1. Survivors—living in chronic pain is hard; it takes bravery, courage, and strength that anyone who has not lived it could never understand.
2. Smart—when the common answers given to a complicated problem like chronic pain are not satisfactory, we

learn to ask more questions, to dig deeper, to become our own researchers and advocates.

I know many chronic pain patients who have become nearly expert at understanding the complexity of their pain in their own search for solutions. They know the drugs, the injections, the therapies, and the approaches that are available because they've tried them or at least researched them. They also know the significant dates and history of how pain came into their lives to rob them. The way that pain blasted down the front door, or crept in slightly at night, came along with someone else (like a seemingly simple injury) and never left, sticking around and robbing them still.

I am confident that if chronic pain is a problem that is affecting your life, you'll understand and appreciate the various aspects of science, healthcare, and business that intersect with it.

That said, some of this information might be more relevant and interesting to you than other information, so to help make it clearer, at the beginning of each chapter, I'll give a quick review of what will be covered. This will allow you to find the topics you are most interested in and what I hope you can get out of it.

First and foremost, this book is for people suffering with

chronic pain and for those that love and care for them. My intention is to bring understanding, hope, and relief to as many people as possible, because ultimately, that is all that matters. Throwing another quasi-effective therapy into the mix or vocalizing an argument for the sake of argument benefits no one. This solution is about restoring people back to life—not just reducing pain, but bringing vitality, productivity, and joy fully back to the lives of those that chronic pain seeks to rob.

It is meant for the many clinical professionals who genuinely care about their patients and want to see them live fuller, happier, pain-free, more productive lives. I hope that you champion the solution and the business case you find presented in this book, and that you see it as valuable and complementary to your work. Indeed, I hope that it allows all of us to more effectively work together at decreasing suffering, improving productivity, and moving towards ever more progressive, safe, and effective therapies.

It is meant for leaders within the medical-industrial complex to enter into the conversation and to be part of the solution that addresses the systemic failings, high costs, and inefficiencies facing our existing global healthcare infrastructure, so that we might deliver better care to those that need it.

It is meant for media and thought leaders throughout the world, so that we can all become champions of innovation to dig deeper and ask the questions to challenge the status quo, resulting in better thinking and a better quality of life for mankind.

I choose to be bold in expressing my view and for making a case for a better solution to chronic pain. Because if I am right—and I have staked my career, reputation, and family's livelihood on the fact that I am, this solution has the potential to help millions of people and the families, friends, and caregivers that surround them.

I am grateful that you've taken the time to read this book and hope that you will find new and helpful information, that you will share this information with others that might benefit from it, and that you'll find ways to join with us in changing the way chronic pain is understood and treated.

CHAPTER 1

A SIMPLE INTRODUCTION TO A COMPLICATED PROBLEM

————

I do not fix problems. I fix my thinking. Then problems fix themselves.

—LOUISE L. HAY

This chapter frames the complicated problem of chronic pain, gives a backstory and history.

I love this quote above by Louise Hay. So much of our problems are problems with our thinking. And so it is with chronic pain. It is possible that everything you think about chronic pain is wrong; everything you've been told or prescribed or tried to treat it with might also be wrong. So, it is my hope that this book will challenge your thinking about chronic pain and the possibility of a better solution to it.

Every single person experiences pain at one point or another; it is something that we know, or think we know, because we've all experienced it—it is part of the human experience. And pain is something we've been conditioned to understand based upon this simple formula: pain = bad, pain = problem. Therefore, the quicker we can mask, dull, or remove the pain, the better. We have been conditioned through our own experiences and social conditioning to think of pain in a cause-and-effect equation. "I feel pain, therefore something is wrong." And sometimes that is the case, but not always, particularly with chronic pain.

So I ask you to suspend what you think you know about chronic pain as we explore it together. I believe that in order for us to fix this problem, we must begin by changing our thinking about it. To change how we think about chronic pain, we must step back, outside of the constraints of existing healthcare delivery, to look independently at the science and to reexamine that science without the pull and biases of current methodologies, economic incentives, and educational and practice disciplines. In other words, we must look at the science independently and approach it in a way that will allow us to use it in crafting a better solution.

Why is that? Because the science has changed. It has changed dramatically in the last few years, so much so that most of the approaches to managing pain are based on antiquated and outdated science and theories. But they continue to be deployed because they get paid for, despite being minimally effective in many cases, and often being risky, dangerous, or addictive—e.g. opioid addiction epidemic.

The latest scientific understanding of pain illustrates clearly that all pain comes from the brain. In fact, the tissues actually have no ability to feel pain; they only have receptors. Those receptors gather information and transmit that information through the nervous system to the brain, which interprets it and generates a sensation or expression of that interpretation. This may seem counterintuitive, because when you put your hand on a hot stove, your hand feels that burning feeling. But the only reason you feel the pain is because you have a brain, not because you have a hand. In this case, as in the case of all acute pain, the pain experience is intended to protect you—to trigger you to take action, e.g. pull your hand off of the hot stove as quickly as possible, to avoid doing more damage to the tissue. In the event that damage to the tissue has occurred, the pain will appropriately linger as the tissue heals and normalizes. Once it's healed, the pain should go away. It is no longer necessary, no longer protective or productive. I have just described acute pain.

Chronic pain is generally accepted to mean that the pain has been present longer than three to six months, which is typically enough time for the tissue to have healed. Chronic pain can also include any pain that is growing disproportionately to the cause, or without a clear cause. In most cases the pain experience of chronic pain is not a protective, productive function, but really just a nuisance, a literal pain.

This pain experience has a top-down impact on the tissues and the body, which are now reacting to this inappropriate expectation of pain that is generated by the brain. The brain is messaging "pain"; the tissues are reacting to that pain expectation and creating a physiological response in the tissue, such as inflammation, limited mobility, increased sensitivity, physiological changes to the nervous system, and so forth. These changes in the tissue create a heightened sensitivity, which then cause normal sensory and movement inputs to be interpreted by the brain falsely as "threats" to which it generates an expanded pain response. It becomes a vicious cycle. If we keep in mind that although the pain is felt in the body, the pain itself is really a product of the brain, we can begin to change our thinking around chronic pain and its treatments.

Is this something you've known? Has a clinician told you about the brain's role in chronic pain or have you read about it in healthcare literature? If the answer is yes, that is great! The next question, then, is: What do we do with this information, how does it change the current course of treatment, or does it affect anything at all? Do we go on just taking drugs to mask it, or pursue therapies that address the tissue solely, even if it's not really the problem? If this is not something that you've been told or read about, or that you knew previously, the reason for it and the answer to how it could or should affect your treatment lies within these pages.

Later in this book, we will get into more details about the disease of chronic pain, and my business partner, David Farley, MD, and I will share a new framework by which we can better understand how chronic pain is more like credit card debt than a cause-and-effect correlation, and solutions to eliminating that "debt." But for now, let's talk about the complicated problem of chronic pain in a broader context.

SIZE AND SCOPE OF THE PROBLEM

It's fairly commonly known and discussed these days that chronic pain affects more people than cancer, diabetes, and cardiovascular disease combined. In the United States, this is more than 100 million people, with similar statistics being reported throughout the world.

The cost of chronic pain is really incalculable, given the

economic burden that arises on an individual, familial, and broader societal level, but it is safe to say that the direct cost of care in treating chronic pain pales in comparison to the real cost imposed on individuals, families, employers, healthcare providers, governments, and society at large.

According to the American Academy of Pain Medicine and others, $600 billion a year is the number thrown around for the financial impact of chronic pain in the United States, as measured by the direct cost of care and the loss of productivity. However, in visiting with many hundreds of chronic pain sufferers about how chronic pain has impacted their lives, it is clear that no price can really be given.

I have been blessed to have a career that has exposed me to and taken me through the range of healthcare approaches from allopathic "Western medicine" to the gamut of "complementary" and "alternative" providers. I grew up in healthcare. My dad was a hospital administrator. I also grew up exposed to alternative care, with an uncle who was a chiropractor. My career has placed me in the operating room with surgeons, in the C-suite of hospitals, and in the private consultation rooms and back offices of private practices owned by MDs, DOs, PhDs, DCs, NDs, PAs, NPs, LAcs, and LMTs, in addition to healers without recognized credentials. Perhaps you, too, in an effort to resolve chronic pain disrupting your life, have been exposed to a broad swath of clinical disciplines.

These career experiences have been eye-opening and profound as I have met many brilliant, caring, and talented clinicians and practitioners. I am honored to know so many devoted professionals. I've been impressed with their dedication, compassion, and contribution. But, systemically, we're failing: failing to be healthier as a whole, failing as a system in solving the more complicated chronic health challenges we face, such as chronic pain. Why is this? With chronic pain, the reasons are varied and complicated; let's walk through them.

WE LOVE PROBLEMS

As a society we *love* discussing problems. Just turn on the radio or TV news, and you'll be bombarded with problems. Many millions of dollars are raised and used in the pursuit of discussing, analyzing, and researching problems. Lucrative careers, billion-dollar companies, and global brands are built on problems. Many seemingly altruistic organizations and feel-good campaigns are designed to bring awareness to problems. At some point, one might wonder, have we lost sight of the goal or misdirected those resources?

What would happen if a cure for a significant disease,

like cancer, was discovered? How would that impact the value of, the investment in, or the perceived contribution of those groups? No doubt "doing good" is the intention, but we should follow the money and ask ourselves if we have allowed the financial incentive of discussing and "researching" solutions to outweigh the value of identifying and building solutions?

Maybe the solutions to many of our most significant killers do exist. There are numerous profound books written. Many caring practitioners are preaching and promoting the prevention and reversal of disease through better habits. Many open-minded individuals are adopting a higher level of ownership in their lives, addressing the growing research on the epigenetics of the body. These are all powerful concepts and empowering solutions for those that seek them, learn them, and adopt them. Exercise, movement, sleep, nutrition, mindfulness, service to others, laughter, joy, etc., all have healing properties. However, generally speaking, they are not institutionally supported or scalable the way a pharmaceutical solution is, for example. Nor are they lucrative to the healthcare institutions that make a lot of money on the research, development, and marketing of healthcare solutions via the mainstream medical establishment.

Shortly before publishing this book, a leak from a Goldman Sachs biotech research report came under fire for asking if "curing patients is a sustainable business model" (April 10, 2018, report entitled "The Genome Revolution"). Indeed, shifts away from any significant industry cause ripples, disruption, and losses for some and gains for the innovator that caused the shift—it's the nature of innovation and disruption.

This is not meant to be an argument against the medical-industrial complex, but we have to look at the whole picture and certainly follow the money when we talk about the many factors to a complicated problem like chronic pain. Without question, health improvements derived by adoption of lifestyle choices at the individual level are not beneficial to the medical-industrial complex as it currently exists.

WHO ARE THE PAIN EXPERTS, REALLY?

In recent years, as my career has shifted to chronic pain, I have attended various conferences on chronic pain and listened to "experts" speak. I have met individually with countless pain management professionals and pain sufferers. From these conversations and experiences, a few other nuances have come to light. The first is that, generally speaking, people don't die from pain—at least not directly. Many people in chronic pain can also suffer from diseases that may be terminal, but pain itself is not really considered a killer. Pain is quite often just something they live with, or at least try to live with.

Consequently, chronic pain does not receive the same levels of funding, research, attention, or discussion as do other diseases. Institutionally, the formal education most physicians and care providers receive about chronic pain is very limited, perhaps even grossly inadequate, and generally related to acute pain or symptomatic pain. New science takes years to filter down through the literature and find its way into medical school textbooks. Practicing physicians typically have to go out of their way to find and really learn the most current changes in any science, especially pain, and then must decide what to do with that info. Does it change their practice?

In all fairness, there are pain specialists, clinicians—typically MDs, DOs, PhDs, or other advanced practitioners—who are board-certified in pain management. But, because pain is such a pervasive problem and often regarded as symptomatic of other conditions, it is nearly impossible to imagine any professional clinician who doesn't in some way treat pain or interact with patients who are in pain.

This fragmentation in pain treatment has only compounded the problem because it has created a scenario where no one really completely "owns" pain management, yet everyone is involved with treating it because his or her patients are inevitably dealing with it. Often clinicians become myopic in their view of the best approach: drug intervention, surgical interventions, various injections, physical manipulation, movement, nutrition, mindfulness, etc. Allopathic or osteopathic pain specialists can be dismissive of chiropractic care, instead recommending drugs, injections, or surgeries. Alternative care providers often promote their approaches of alignment, movement, nutrition, sleep, and mindfulness over the quick fix of a pill or injection, and have been doing so tirelessly since long before anyone realized we had developed an opioid addiction epidemic.

And yet, all of these professionals will probably admit that their solution or approach to chronic pain is, in truth, inadequate.

The acknowledgment of the inadequacies of any single solution to chronic pain has led to the establishment of multidisciplinary approaches, where multiple clinical modalities are brought together in an effort to treat chronic pain. Given the complexity of pain, this is a sensible approach, and I applaud and honor the collaboration. Truthfully, more interdisciplinary collaboration is needed in healthcare. Yet the problem continues and, ultimately, the cost and impact of chronic pain grows. Perhaps this is due to the fact that, ultimately, each of these solutions, whether delivered individually, consecutively, or concurrently, is inadequate and slightly misdirected.

Chronic pain is a disease. But, as mentioned previously, because people don't die from it, it has received minuscule research investment. Much of the research and training on chronic pain is funded by pharmaceutical companies who may not have an overriding interest in maintaining neutrality. Pain education receives too little formal training and discussion in medical schools and other professional education. And what education is given is primarily related to acute pain, not chronic pain, and is based on outdated theories and models. The latest scientific research on chronic pain has revealed chronic pain to be a problem of the brain, yet most of the therapies address only the tissue or are a drug with impact to the entire chemistry of the body.

Pioneering researchers and clinicians, such as Lorimer Moseley, David Butler, Adriaan Louw, Norman Doidge, and others, have been an important yet minority voice in explaining that chronic pain is a problem of the brain.

Neuroscientists now know that in chronic pain, the brain becomes fixated on and "wired" to expect pain. It has less to do with the tissues in which the pain is being felt, even when there was initially or even continues to be some pathology or trauma in the tissue, and is more about the brain's expectation of pain. Since the brain expects the pain, the body and tissues react, and we have the beginning of what becomes a very vicious loop of pain expectation and body systems reaction, each feeding on the other.

This perpetual chicken-and-egg dilemma feeds into the turf war of who owns the management of chronic pain. Pharmaceutical approaches, surgery, injections, stem cells, biologics, physical manipulation, movement, nutrition, sleep, mindfulness, cognitive behavioral therapy, and more all provide some relief. Many of these are often inadequate, incomplete, or not lasting. As professionals and patients realize that these approaches are not consistently or wholly effective, unintentionally, the conversation for the sufferer moves towards resignation. Our chronic pain sufferer is left to either accept a life of pain or continue on an endless journey of mediocre therapies.

PAIN SUFFERERS BECOME MORE COMPLICATED

As a chronic pain sufferer, or as someone who cares for a chronic pain sufferer, you know that chronic pain is very complicated, very individual, and even very subjective. Likely, you've lived through the inevitable evolution: when one approach does not work, you move to the next. In time, for many patients, due to the process of disappointing outcome after disappointing outcome, chronic pain begins to take on an emotional component that only makes the situation worse. Discouragement, depression, and anxiety often add fuel to an already growing fire. Sometimes, this is exacerbated by how patients and clinicians alike interact in growing frustration over limited outcomes and few options. In some cases, it is also possible that the emotions themselves contribute to or cause pain.

The condition of chronic pain sufferers, when faced with months, years, or decades of chronic pain, often becomes increasingly complicated as they develop comorbidities and side effects. Because they hurt, they move less, becoming increasingly sedentary. Sleep is compromised. The common side effect of weight gain adds more burden to an already strained and hurting body. This is compounded further by increased mental anguish, isolation, and limitation from a life they would otherwise love to be living.

Medications may, particularly over the long term, make this cascade of decline even more profound. Medications can cause cognitive impairment, disrupted sleep, constipation or compromised digestion, and the feeling of just being numbed out. This often leads chronic pain sufferers to begin feeling, to some degree or another, trapped in their bodies, caged by a life that they would have never chosen, and angry that no one, nothing, has helped. Has this been your case or the case of someone you care for? If so, I am sorry, and please know you are not alone.

DISRUPTION DISRUPTS THE STATUS QUO

What if there was a solution to address the root cause of chronic pain—the brain? What if the brain of the chronic pain sufferer could be hacked, reprogrammed, rewired, and restored to a more normalized perception of the pain response in the body? What if that solution required no drugs, needles, or surgery? What if that solution was safe, consistently effective, and totally noninvasive?

Would it change the world? Would it improve and save millions of lives?

Or would it be ignored because those "in the know" do not understand it? Would it be ridiculed and dismissed as "too good to be true"? Would it be diminished because it does not fit or fully integrate into any of the existing professional infrastructure? Might the economics of *resolving* chronic pain threaten the economics of *treating* chronic pain?

The good news for anyone who is dealing with chronic pain or those who love someone in chronic pain is that such a solution does exist. Is it perfect? No. But it is the safest, most consistently effective and appealing therapy for chronic pain. And if it can be successfully understood, properly adopted, and capitalized, it can change the world and many millions of lives along the way.

These following chapters will discuss this therapy in greater detail. I will give a review of its origin and history and explain, in fairly basic terms, its mechanism of action and its fundamental approach. I will explain why most people and most professionals haven't heard of this approach and, if they have, why they may not understand it. I will walk through the market factors and conditions that have created barriers to effective commercialization and the steps my partners and I have taken to overcome those barriers. I will share my vision for the development of this therapy throughout North America and the world. And I will make a case for a better solution to the epidemic of chronic pain.

CHAPTER 2

THE COMPLICATED CONTEXT OF CHRONIC PAIN

———

For me context is the key—from that comes the understanding of everything.

—KENNETH NOLAND

This chapter gives the context of understanding how chronic pain has been understood and treated historically and suggests why this context creates limitations in adequately addressing it.

Context matters. The context of understanding, treating, and deploying solutions to chronic pain is complicated and fragmented. Another important aspect to context is authorship or voice. The party or parties with the most clout, the greatest reputation, and often the biggest bank accounts write the dominant narrative of any story, and about any industry. Context frames credibility. So, for healthcare, the medical-industrial complex, supported in large measure by pharmaceutical companies, tells the story that the masses hear the most.

Institutional healthcare is big business—an intelligent and sophisticated business that has effectively conditioned healthcare consumers to believe that for most maladies there is a pill for this, a quick fix for that. Even for the terminal and chronic illness, the recommended protocols are usually pharmaceutical and surgical. It is the expected approach, accepted as the valid approach, and the overarching standard of professional care.

Certainly, pharmaceutical solutions can be very helpful, and for many conditions surgical approaches may be necessary. But the point is the "medical establishment" and healthcare consumers are conditioned to trust this authority because it is the only authority we know. Complementary and alternative care, and personal ownership for choosing a healthy lifestyle, are small medicine, not big medicine. These approaches, even if safer, even if more healthful, are not as lucrative as and certainly not scalable like those of Big Pharma and the large medical infrastructure we have built over decades. Indeed, capitalism, and I say this as a capitalist, has shaped the evolution of healthcare globally, and certainly in North America. I think most would accept this. However, perhaps more controversial would be to suggest that not only has capitalism shaped the evolution of the institution, but also the players within it.

THE ALLOPATHIC APPROACH

"Do no harm" is the oath all physicians ascribe to. Indeed, physicians devote their lives to serving, helping, and healing; this is in no way a suggestion to the contrary. But doctors are also human, subject to the influence of others, mentors, peers, environments, marketers, and their own internal biases, the same as anyone.

Medical school is exceptionally rigorous, residency worse. By design, it prepares, strengthens, and indoctrinates its pupils with the knowledge they need to practice medicine with exactness, authority, and confidence, according to their field. But let me suggest that perhaps this exacting and refining process of developing someone into a medical doctor may create some flaws that are potentially harmful, at least when it comes to understanding and treating chronic pain.

Most physicians receive very little training in medical school about pain, and what they do receive is predominately related to acute pain. Additionally, physicians, at least in the US, are trained in biochemistry. This is required coursework, and rightfully so, given that most will be prescribing drugs and need to be knowledgeable about chemistry and about the biochemical mechanism of action of those drugs in the body. This focus on biochemistry shades many physicians' vision of the body, disease, and treatments. I also suggest that due to the breadth and depth of knowledge they acquire in their training, and the rigor, demands, and length of the process in which physicians are prepared, they are typically confident (in some cases even arrogant).

Of course, this is a gross generality. But my point is that this level of absolute preparation creates the risk of being myopic—seeing the world, seeing disease, seeing care through the lens of a certain discipline and having belief that it is rooted in the absolute best science and understanding. Historically, we have witnessed a vast dichotomy between allopathic and alternative care, which stems from this type of thinking. Fortunately, this is changing, as we see not only warmer regard amongst the disciplines of care, but an increasing number of integrated healthcare practices.

For most MDs, the approach to treating chronic pain starts with a prescription, moves to injections, and then is followed by surgical interventions, as each stage proves incomplete in resolving the chronic pain. A common prescribing approach has been to continually up the dosage on a particular medication until one of two things happens: one, the pain goes away, or two, the side effects become too intolerable. Some, perhaps a growing number, are now recommending complementary therapies, but the institutional approach is and certainly has been pharmacological, followed by increasingly invasive procedures.

With a training background rooted in biochemistry, and heavy influence from pharmaceutical marketing (both direct-to-consumer advertising and sales reps), pharmaceutical drugs have been the staple initial approach for treating chronic pain. Again, this is affected by context—namely, by a consumer perspective that drugs are the solution: an appetite for a quick and easy fix versus implementing a higher level of ownership with a discipline to exercise, eat better, sleep more, reduce stress, etc., and our own human history of substance use, going back to early man's use of opium, alcohol, or other chemicals to reduce pain (temporarily).

Secondarily, physician practices have, by necessity, turned to a throughput model; doctors have less time with patients than they would like. The origin, history, and mechanics of pain can be difficult to understand and often, particularly in acute pain, the pain will resolve on its own, as it should. So, a drug, particularly an opioid, has been an effective short-term strategy and quick solution. The problem occurs when the short-term strategy is used long term, and opioids unintentionally become the go-to long-term solution.

More will be discussed about opioids as well as the neuroleptic and anticonvulsant drugs and other therapies later in the book.

I think it's safe to say that given the high rate of opioid addiction now burdening families, communities, and institutions across the country (and throughout the world), the opioids were not and are not the right solution to chronic pain. It is worth suggesting that it is not just that opioids weren't the right solution, but perhaps it was the thinking and the behavior framed within the institution of healthcare today that allowed them to become the flawed solution. We should believe that doctors have acted with the best intentions prescribing these drugs—they don't need to be vilified. However, we should recognize that a system that can facilitate caring people, who have vowed to do no harm, to produce this much harm, is perhaps flawed, fallible, and imperfect.

THE ALTERNATIVE CARE APPROACH

The alternative care practitioners offer a different conundrum when it comes to addressing chronic pain. Having grown up with chiropractic care and, just as influentially, having spent several years interacting professionally with a broad range of clinicians across the spectrum of "alternative medicine," I have a great respect for the work they do, particularly the early pioneers. Progressive thinking should always be championed. The work of many of these practitioners is pioneering. These clinicians have historically been diminished by the healthcare mainstream and labeled wacky, hippy, voodoo, old-world, and more, yet they have persisted and grown, while quietly delivering their care patient by patient. The wisdom of their practices—movement, nutrition, sleep, mindfulness, energy, balancing the body systems—has slowly begun to gain favor amongst healthcare consumers. Many have turned to these practices after not finding adequate solutions to their health problems through biomedical means. This is certainly true with chronic pain sufferers.

Greater discussion about and exploration of the history and the latest understanding of chronic pain will be presented later. Because chronic pain hurts, it begins to have influence and impact on many areas of health: activity level, mood, energy, sleep, appetite, digestion, and weight control. Sometimes pharmaceutical drugs will make these things worse. Perhaps an injury was the initial cause, but when the pain becomes chronic—in other words, the pain didn't resolve in the normal or expected timeframe—the person would likely benefit from practices that don't just mask the pain, but that get the person moving better, sleeping better, absorbing more nutrition, reducing inflammation, and changing their attitude towards this pain experience. The range of what alternative-care providers can and do offer is a valuable contribution in addressing these issues more wholly and more holistically.

The problems with alternative care from an institutional standpoint are:

- Alternative care usually takes more time. Because it is often very hands on, it requires more time from both the patient and the care provider.
- This type of care is less economically advantageous for the provider because, historically, it has not usually been reimbursed by insurance, although this is changing in some parts of the country and for some types of care.
- Alternative care is often not scalable, even within the same discipline (I have heard numerous chiropractors state that the biggest problem with and threat to their profession is other chiropractors). There is a consistency and scalability in Western institutional healthcare, underlined by the use of pharmaceuticals, that is hard to replicate across a fragmented and varied body of alternative-care providers.

The problem with alternative care from a patient perspective is varied:

- First, access—finding and accessing the right practitioner, both from a discipline standpoint as well as quality of care standpoint, can be problematic. Again, solutions and quality are often not consistent even within same discipline.
- Second, time and engagement are on a longer scale. Healing holistically is not usually an immediate solution, even if it is better. It requires commitment on the part of the patient, which often necessitates the patient make changes in their life that are not easy. As a society, we've been conditioned to seek the quick fix, the easy cure, rather than embrace the struggle and commitment of choosing health through our lifestyle—eating right, exercising, managing stress, etc.
- Finally, the cost of "alternative care" is often completely out of pocket. And while an investment in one's health is arguably the best investment someone can make, much like the ease of pills, we've been conditioned to expect insurance coverage. When something is not covered by insurance, we can find ourselves assuming a lack of validity of the treatment.

So, neither camp of care has the perfect solution. Neither is perfectly suited to address the epidemic of chronic pain both consistently and effectively without some risks, complications, or challenges. Yet both certainly have many great things to offer, and discussing them helps frame the canvas of understanding as I paint the picture of the complexity of solving the problem of chronic pain.

FOLLOW THE MONEY

Another context that is critical to consider is that of money: how the economics of care shape, influence, and drive clinical considerations for providers and patients. Later on, we'll explore the economic drivers of each approach to treating chronic pain, procedure by procedure, but here let me just state the obvious—the economics of healthcare today are a mess, a deep mess. The insurance reimbursement/insurance coverage model has distorted the reality of effective healthcare economics. Costs have been over-inflated in many cases, while simultaneously patients have lost sight of value. Plenty could and really should be written about the history and evolution of healthcare economics in the United States, and I don't purport to have a solution to that globally, although I think any solution that lacks these three things at the consumer level will inevitably fail:

Access—Patients need access to affordable, productive, preventatively leaning care. No doubt there is currently a vast difference in access to quality care based upon personal economic circumstances. Access is vitally important, but a shift towards prevention could improve quality outcomes significantly and greatly reduce the costs associated with treating disease, particularly the heavy costs of "lifestyle diseases" related to weight gain, dietary and fitness decline, and stress/mind management. This comes from improved access and better education.

Education—Somewhere along the way, as a society, we've lost the inclination towards health education. Literally, we've forgotten how to live healthily. If we haven't forgotten that we should, we've probably forgotten how, and certainly forgotten the joy in living healthily. We don't even have physical education (PE) in schools anymore. Even recesses and play times are being shortened, with the government spending money trying to motivate youth to move for at least sixty minutes a day.

We all could benefit from better understanding, better information, better tools, and even better access to empower ourselves to choose health daily—long before we are sick.

Accountability—Access and education are both necessary, but there has to be a higher level of accountability built into a disruptive healthcare payer system. If people are more inclined to make healthy choices, they cost less to care for long-term. When people chronically abuse themselves with bad choices, they inevitably develop disease(s) and cost more to care for. Better healthcare must include access to resources and education about why and how to live healthier. It should also include some driver(s) of accountability, probably financially, to align the individual with the cost and deliverable for the whole of healthcare delivery. A lack of alignment in (any of) these areas will inevitably result in imbalance and dysfunction in cost of care or access to care.

Access, education, and accountability are necessary because they reinfuse ownership and rebalance the power of healing between patient and provider. Seeing these aspects as fundamental is necessary to building a better healthcare business and, quite frankly, the future of healthcare in general. These are considerations we've factored in as we've built our business model, which we'll discuss in greater detail later in the book.

Now, let's understand what has happened to clinical practice over the last decade or two.

Insurance reimbursements (what doctors get paid for procedures) have been in decline for decades. This means doctors are making less money—less money for the same procedures they have been doing for years. Simultaneously to revenues declining, costs have been increasing. Operating costs are increasing, due in large part to the cumbersome process of dealing with insurance. It is a burden to have to contract and negotiate with insurance companies on the front end, and requires a significant ongoing operating cost to manage the process: receive prior authorization, submit (and often resubmit) the bill, and chase the money to ensure payment. The previously healthy operating margin afforded to private practice has been greatly eroded.

To make up this lost margin, and as a product of the fact that more people are insured (and sicker), most practices have adopted a throughput model. It is now a volume business, and the result is very few minutes with the doctor and often declining quality of care. To manage this volume, practices employ more nurses, medical assistants, and mid-level providers, all of which translates to increased cost burden and less profitability.

Consequently, we see private practices banding together to create "large groups" in an effort to try to create some operating efficiencies, share resources, and create stronger negotiating power with the insurance payers. Or we see the practices selling to hospitals to offload most of the administrative burden they face—in some places, we see significant pressure on the part of payers and hospitals to drive this consolidation. Ultimately, in many cases, the quality of care is affected, and the stress level of the practitioners increased. These realities further erode the viability of finding, placing, or growing disruption and novel approaches to care (particularly for chronic pain) because the bandwidth and operating reality just don't allow it.

MY UNIQUE PERSPECTIVE

The last context I want to share is my own because I think it has had great influence on how I saw the problem of chronic pain and how I saw and modeled a novel solution to that problem. As mentioned previously, when I was a kid, my dad was in hospital administration. I have fond memories of going to the hospitals where he worked, meeting the doctors, and being in that environment. I also had an uncle who was a chiropractor, so I grew up getting chiropractic adjustments. Though he didn't promote many of the nutritional and functional programs that many DCs do now, it gave me a broader exposure that I might not have had otherwise, and probably primed me for the work I did later in my career with functional medicine providers across the gamut of disciplines.

My first job after completing an MBA was working in hospital marketing, which furthered my exposure to healthcare and deepened my understanding of the drivers of care at that level. I went on to work in the sleep medicine industry in the mid-2000s—around the height of the boom for sleep awareness, sleep labs, and a thrust to greater analysis of sleep disorders and related comorbidities. This was also a period of consolidation and economic change that ultimately led to a shift away from sleep labs to home sleep studies, but left more people aware of and addressing sleep disorders, and further exposed me to the business and economic drivers of healthcare.

For the following nearly ten years, I went to work in the hearing aid industry. I had the privilege of working with and contributing to two growth-award companies (*Inc.* magazine and *Portland Business Journal*) in this space and learned intimately the drivers of successful clinical practice. Hearing aids however, are typically not covered by insurance—they are an out-of-pocket expense—and they are not inexpensive (the average sales price is around $6,000 for a set). Beyond hearing aids, I had experience adding other ancillary, often cash-model, revenue procedures or products to clinics in an effort to help these physicians offset the declining insurance reimbursements they faced in their normal procedural offerings. This experience of helping clinicians improve their business operations, refine their marketing, and sharpen their selling processes was profound—and would later serve as a critical experience and the predicate business model upon which we modeled our chronic pain solution.

During most of these years, my wife battled her own chronic health conditions, from which she found little relief though biomedical care. Disappointed with the options of drugs or traditional care, she turned to alternative medicine, and over the years saw dozens of clinicians in all disciplines of care: chiropractors, naturopaths, acupuncturists, herbalists, functional medicine doctors, counselors, meditation gurus, and many others, some of whom have no formal credentials. It was in the midst of this period when I had the opportunity to go to work for a medical device start-up, which had a breath test to measure oxidative stress (i.e. free-radical damage).

This device was an alternative to blood or urinalysis assays and a more convenient and cost-effective way to measure oxidative stress changes that could result from lifestyle changes such as diet, exercise, sleep, stress management, etc. Over the three years working with this technology, coupled with my wife's health journey, I deepened my exposure to, knowledge of, and appreciation for these types of care providers. Yet I was struck by the variance in approaches, and sometimes thoroughness of clinicians, even within the same discipline.

Ultimately, my wife found healing through a different alternative healing modality called the Dynamic Neural Retraining System (DNRS), but this experience of personally and professionally interacting with so many different types of clinicians across every discipline was valuable. It exposed me to so much of their thinking, modalities, and philosophies of care, and on a personal level helped me understand the emotional, intellectual, and physical toll that it places on individuals who can't find solutions to their complicated health problems—despite visiting so many (usually very caring) practitioners. All of this process and history, I believe, uniquely prepared me to see the chronic pain problem differently and to have the context to prepare a better solution.

Indeed, context matters.

CHAPTER 3

THE GENESIS, BIRTH, AND NEAR DEATH OF A NOVEL THERAPY

We can't solve problems by using the same kind of thinking we used when we created them.

—ALBERT EINSTEIN

This chapter discusses the origin of new medical technology for treating chronic pain and explains why this technology didn't immediately take off. It gets into the medical aspects of pain, this particular approach, and David Farley, MD, explains the technology and pain management from the perspective of a physician.

In 2011, I was working as director of sales and marketing

for a medical device company in the wellness, prevention, and anti-aging industry—our main product was a diagnostic to measure oxidative stress, more commonly known as free-radical damage. I had helped the company put the "go-to-market" strategy together, launch, and build the initial sales channels. The sales focus was on wellness, anti-aging, and preventative medicine practitioners. The earliest adopters of this technology were chiropractors, being both comfortable with cash-model and instrument-oriented therapies. The marketing of the technology also put me in contact with progressively thinking MDs, naturopaths, and many other clinicians. I traveled the world representing the technology at regional conferences and large events like Wright/Gaby, American Academy of Anti-Aging Medicine (A4M), and MEDICA, one of the largest medical device conferences in the world, held in Düsseldorf, Germany.

It was during this time that I became aware of a technology known in the FDA paperwork and the medical literature as Scrambler Therapy (ST). Scrambler Therapy was purported to be a new and novel way to treat chronic pain by retraining the brain noninvasively and without drugs, needles, surgery, or side effects. This ST technology was, at this time, being traditionally marketed, as most medical devices are, through a selling model to clinicians. Through a family contact that had secured the rights to the ST market in the western US, I was able to create a sub-dealer opportunity under them to sell and market the device.

Believing that a noninvasive, nonpharmacological solution to chronic pain could be a game changer, I began to devote time, energy, resources, and money into efforts to market the therapy. I called on doctors, mostly MDs and DOs. I booked exhibitor booths and attended pain conferences. I went to my network of medical contacts.

The common response, however, was a mix of amused curiosity, a look of incredulity, or outright dismissal. Rightly so; the medical professionals I spoke with wanted to know things that I and the company couldn't fully or accurately answer, particularly from their standpoint of having a basis of knowledge that didn't fully support the underlying theories and mechanism of action of the technology. Most physicians were taught something called the Gate Control Theory of pain, which was published in the 1960s—old science (more on that later in the chapter). They wanted to know how it worked and how it differed from other electrical stimulation technologies like TENS, micro-current, or other electrical stimulation therapies. They wanted to understand its mechanism of action and the exact electrical neuromodulation output it generated. They wanted studies, and the limited pilot studies that had been completed at the Mayo Clinic and Johns Hopkins University were not sufficient for their needs. They wanted double-blind, placebo-controlled studies with longitudinal outcomes for fifteen years. They wanted published peer-reviewed journal articles. And it seemed at times that they wanted blood.

It seemed I had trespassed in holy lands, blasphemed a medical deity, and insulted the doctors' intelligence.

Frequently I was told directly, or implicitly, that I was wasting their time (and mine) with "snake oil," that this was nothing new and likely nothing novel or effective at creating a lasting result. I heard repeated things like "No way can you create durable (lasting) relief without some sort of drug intervention," and other comments along these lines. Occasionally, I had a positive, engaged, and optimistic dialogue with a clinician, in which they expressed a genuine inquisitiveness. A few times, they did have enough optimism that I was asked to schedule a next-step dialogue, or to book a "demo" of the technology.

When this occasion presented itself, it was cause for excitement, because it was not often. My colleagues in the distributorship would fly in to participate, providing a slightly deeper level of understanding or discussion points, and running a day or two of no-cost demo treatments on the patients of the interested doctor. Almost universally, patients treated in these no-cost demos saw relief, sometimes substantial or even total relief.

Many times, the doctors were impressed with the results they saw, though they seemed a bit disbelieving about its mechanisms of action. Unfortunately, far more often than not, interest would be killed when we'd start talking about the process, price, and economics of buying the technology. Because of the high price point of the technology and lack of insurance reimbursement, coupled with limited understanding of how it worked mechanically or in the body (by both the medical community and the company selling the technology) very few devices were sold nationwide or globally.

UNDERSTANDING PAIN

Before we get into the next phase of relevant experience and learning what ultimately would evolve into the business concept that we have now with Radiant, I have asked David Farley, MD, my cofounder and the chief medical officer of Radiant Pain Relief Centres, to explain in greater detail chronic pain and his history with Scrambler Therapy (ST); take a deeper dive into the history and origin of the technology and its mechanism of action; as well as color the circumstances of chronic pain and its management from the standpoint of a physician.

Dave is a very warm, delightful doctor, who cares deeply for his patients. He is also very bright. A valedictorian in his undergrad class at Brigham Young University, he went on to a joint medical school program at Harvard Medical School and MIT. Through his clinical exposure in residency, he developed a deep love for clinical practice, and chose to go into family medicine over research or other medical specialties that would have certainly been available to a person of his intellect and training. Dave has operated a highly successful private-practice family medicine business in West Linn, a bedroom community suburb of Portland, Oregon, for thirty years. During that time, Dave has cared for thousands across all ages, treating patients from pregnancy and childbirth through end-of-life care.

INVESTIGATING SCRAMBLER THERAPY

When I was first introduced to Scrambler Therapy by Brendon Lundberg in 2013, being the skeptical physician that I am, I was not interested, feeling that it sounded too good to be true. However, my dissatisfaction with the therapy options for chronic pain (neuropathic pain in particular) pushed me to look into it. The obvious question was: "How could something supposedly so effective be so obscure?" But Brendon encouraged me to at least look at the studies that had come out of Johns Hopkins and the Mayo Clinic.

Although, in the US, most of the studies have been done by Thomas J. Smith at Johns Hopkins and Charles Loprinzi at the Mayo Clinic, there were some problems. First, all of the studies to date have been small pilot studies, and second, there are really no placebo-controlled trials.

I first reviewed an article by Thomas J. Smith, MD, the Harry J. Duffey Family Professor of Palliative Medicine at Johns Hopkins Medical School, that was published in the *Journal of Pain and Symptom Management* in January 2012.[1] Although the study was small and considered a pilot study, I was very impressed by the quality of the study design and even more impressed by the results. Basically, they found a 91% reduction in pain with Scrambler Therapy

---

1   G. Marineo et al., "Scrambler Therapy May Relieve Chronic Neuropathic Pain More Effectively Than Guideline-Based Drug Management: Results of a Pilot, Randomized, Controlled Trial," *Journal of Pain and Symptom Management* 43, no. 1 (2012): 87–95.

versus a 28% reduction with standard drug therapy. That is a P value of <0.0001, impressive by anyone's standards.

Dr. Smith followed with a study of a condition that has been a nightmare for all of us treating chronic pain, a condition known as postherpetic neuralgia (PHN), commonly called post-shingles pain. In this small study,[2] ten patients with postherpetic neuralgia were treated with ten sessions of Scrambler Therapy and dropped their VAS pain score from 7.64 ± 1.46 to 0.42 ± 0.89, a 95% reduction in pain. Pain relief continued at two- and three-month assessments. Despite the small number, anyone who has treated any number of PHN patients will recognize the significance of this.

Charles Loprinzi, MD, is the Regus Professor of Breast Cancer Research at the Mayo Clinic. Although Dr. Loprinzi had not yet published anything on his Scrambler Therapy Research, I had heard that he was just winding up a study on Scrambler Therapy on chemotherapy-induced peripheral neuropathy (CIPN). Loprinzi had a reputation for being very skeptical and never shied away from publishing negative reports. In fact, it was his group that did the study showing that gabapentin was no better than a placebo in treating CIPN.[3] I called Dr. Loprinzi and had

2 T. J. Smith and G. Marineo, "Treatment of Postherpetic Pain with Scrambler Therapy, a Patient-specific Neurocutaneous Electrical Stimulation Device," *American Journal of Hospice & Palliative Care* 35, no. 5 (2013): 812–813.

3 R. D. Rao et al., "Efficacy of Gabapentin in the Management of Chemotherapy-induced Peripheral Neuropathy," *Cancer* 110, no. 9 (2007): 2110–2118.

a very interesting discussion with him. He told me of the extremely positive results they were getting in CIPN using ST, which eventually was published in *Supportive Care in Cancer*.[4] There was a 53% reduction in pain, 44% reduction in tingling, and 37% reduction in numbness that lasted throughout the ten-week follow-up. Again, anyone who treats CIPN will recognize the significance of this. After this discussion, I went back to Brendon and told him that I felt an obligation to my patients to give it a try.

In October of 2013, Brendon and I arranged to have a Scrambler Therapy device brought to my office where we did "demo" treatments on twenty-five of my chronic pain patients over a three-day period of time. Like most doctors, I am quite skeptical about new therapies, so I was astonished at the results we had. Most of the patients treated had been my patients for years or decades, and I knew them well. I have to admit that I was stunned at the results. Many of the patients left my clinic pain-free, not being able to remember the last time they had been pain-free. So that is how it all began for me, with so many patients that I had known for years leaving my office pain-free for the first time that they could remember. It was then obvious to me that we needed to pursue this and prove to ourselves the effectiveness of Scrambler Therapy.

---

4   D. R. Pachman et al., "Pilot Evaluation of Scrambler Therapy for the Treatment of Chemotherapy-induced Peripheral Neuropathy," *Supportive Care in Cancer* 23, no. 4 (2007): 943–951.

Because we have been treating patients full-time since early 2014, I have come to understand why the research has been limited. The cost of funding trials has been a limiter, with neither the inventor nor the previous licensee having the capital to fund any large studies. The reason there are no placebo-controlled trials is because of the nature of the treatment process. There are people trying to come up with a sham device, but in my opinion, a true placebo-controlled trial is not feasible because of the nature of the treatment process.

In order to properly treat a patient with ST, you have to have proper lead placement. In order to get proper lead placement, you have to have continual feedback from the patient regarding very specific sensations with the initiation of treatment. If you don't get that initial feedback, you turn off the device, reposition the leads and try again until you achieve the specifics that indicate lead placement is correct. I believe this process prohibits a true blinded, placebo-controlled trial. There are just certain procedures that are not amenable to placebo control. Laparoscopic versus open-colon surgery is a classic example, as would be childbirth. For nearly all procedures, outcomes generally improve through repetition—the more you do them, the more consistently positive the results become. The same is true with ST.

I have been pushing for more randomized studies that

compare Scrambler Therapy to other widely recognized current standard therapies, rather than placebo. Thomas J. Smith at Johns Hopkins did such a study, referenced in the footnotes. In it, he compared ST to standard guideline-directed drug therapy in three types of chronic neuropathic pain: 1) post-surgical neuropathic pain, 2) postherpetic neuralgia, and 3) spinal stenosis-related neuropathic pain. If you look at the study, you will see that it was randomized very well. Consistent with the experience of all of us who have treated chronic pain with medications, the guideline-directed drug therapy control group's response was unimpressive and they only dropped their VAS pain score from 8.1 to 5.8 (a 28% reduction in pain), and this remained quite steady throughout the three-month follow-up period. However, the Scrambler Therapy group had their VAS score reduced from 8.0 to 0.7 (a 90% reduction in pain), and this only rebounded to a VAS score of 2.0 at three months. This was true for all three types of neuropathic pain.

This is very consistent with our experience at Radiant. We have not done any prospective studies, but in tracking our patient results with all types of chronic pain, we have achieved an average of 84% reduction in pain and nearly 90% of our patients get their VAS score to 0 or 1.0. This relief can last anywhere from thirty days to indefinitely. For those who have a recurrence of their pain, one or two "booster" treatments will usually get them back out of pain.

There are further studies being done at Johns Hopkins, Mayo, and elsewhere. There is no question in my mind that this will not be an obscure therapy in a relatively short period of time.

To better understand why this is, it is important to understand pain—chronic pain in particular.

CHRONIC PAIN PHYSIOLOGY

Pain is typically divided into two categories: acute and chronic. Acute pain is physiologic and has a protective role in preventing further injury. When you place your hand on a hot stove, the burn hurts, so you will immediately remove your hand to avoid further injury. Likewise, when we sprain an ankle, the pain from the injury discourages us from walking or running on it and causing more damage to the tissue. On the other hand, chronic pain (typically defined as pain lasting longer than three to six months) is often pathologic, meaning that the protective, physiologic role is no longer operative and a vicious cycle of inappropriate nerve signaling and brain processing results in the perception of persistent pain long after the protective role of the pain has passed.

For example, if a person herniates a disc in the lumbar spine, scar tissue will typically form around the disc herniation within three to six months and protect the disc from further herniation, yet pain can persist indefinitely in some cases. Another example is phantom limb pain. If someone has a finger amputated by a table saw (not a recommended activity), the stump of the amputated digit would typically heal in two to three months. However, the perception of pain in the no-longer-existing phalanx can continue to cause pain for years and, again, sometimes indefinitely. Let's take the ankle sprain mentioned earlier. Most sprains, even severe ones (grade III) will completely heal in six to twelve weeks. However, in a small percentage of cases, the injury can lead to a chronic pain condition known as complex regional pain syndrome (CRPS), a particularly challenging chronic pain condition that has been baffling medical professionals for decades.

NEW PAIN SCIENCE

Since 1965, when Melzack and Wall published their landmark paper, the Gate Control Theory of pain has been the basis of nearly all research on pain and its treatment.[5] While this has been quite acceptable and explanatory for acute pain, as the inventor of Scrambler Therapy, Professor Giuseppe Marineo, explains:

> [The Gate Control Theory] has significant limitations concerning the analytical representation of chronic

---

5   R. Melzack and P. D. Wall, "Pain Mechanisms: A New Theory," Science 150, no. 699 (1965): 971–979.

pain in its various neurological and pathological mechanisms. The most significant observed gap is that while this theory can interpret 'mechanical' pain transmission methods, it cannot interpret properties of the associated information, such as emerging properties and pain response in the most elevated and complex systems such as memory and learning. These responses are non-linear and dynamically variable through time, compared to the pain stimulus itself."[6]

In other words, chronic pain does not usually have any correlation to the tissue any longer—it grows in duration of presence, sticking around longer than would be appropriate or growing disproportionately to the cause, or in some cases of chronic pain, without a clear cause. This is supported by the latest scientific understanding of pain. In fact, in 1999 Melzack published a new theory called the Pain Neuromatrix, which has since been evolved to be known as the Threat Neuromatrix.

The Threat Neuromatrix model involves a complex association of experiences across multiple brain areas, designed to "protect" a person from threat by hardwiring certain response patterns to stimuli in an effort to create a more effective response to threats in the environment. Essentially these are "learned" responses to certain stimuli.

---

6   "Scrambler Therapy Theory Bases," http://www.scramblertherapy.org/scrambler-therapy-theory-bases.htm

CHRONIC PAIN IS LIKE CREDIT CARD DEBT

Brendon here again, to break this down a bit more. Like the saying "We do not see the world as it is; we see it as we are," the human brain adapts to experiences as well as other factors such as beliefs, cultural factors, environment, and expectation. It filters all sensory inputs from the body and its surroundings through these filters of experience, to assign meaning and create an interpretation which triggers an action or a response. In essence, pain is a response mechanism to trigger action. In chronic pain, the brain has become "wired" to interpret more sensations as threats than is optimal, resulting in hypersensitivity and an increased pain response in the body. This is a result not just of tissue trauma, but of an accumulation of "threats." So essentially, we don't feel pain as it is; we feel it as we are.

We tend to think of pain as having a direct correlation to tissue trauma or injury, and see pain as an indication of something wrong in the tissue. It is better to think of it as an action indicator, particularly in chronic pain, indicating that the body has accumulated and not effectively processed, too many threat experiences and is not responding appropriately to its sensory inputs any longer.

Think of this as credit card debt. If you have a card with, say, a $3,000 credit limit and you use it routinely for groceries, gas, school supplies for the kids, and weekends away, it's no big deal as long as you're making at least the minimum payments. But if, all of a sudden, the car breaks down and you have a $1,300 car repair bill, but you had $2,000 of previous charges still on the credit balance, this is a problem. You have now exceeded the credit limit. This means penalties—over-limit fees. Plus, how are you going to buy groceries when you don't get paid for four more days? And what about the kids' soccer registration? What were once routine, innocuous charges have now become a very "painful" situation.

We might look at the car breaking down as the cause of this "pain," but in fact, it is the accumulation of many charges, credit left on the balance, and the car repair that make it "hurt" so much. And it hurts a lot worse because of what else it costs you: the ability to use it to buy groceries or pay for the soccer registration. If someone is accumulating debt and not paying it off, the debt remains. The same is true in the body. A trauma of some sort may be the reason that a person has been pushed to or beyond their "threat debt limit," resulting in pain, but had there been less debt on the balance before the traumatic event, it may not have resulted in such a painful experience. If the pain is preventing or limiting other important life functions, it can actually make the pain worse.

It seems that, due to various factors (genetics, lifestyle, habits, environment), some people may have lower "threat debt limits," meaning that they have a lower threshold for what will cause them to hit or exceed that limit, resulting in a maladaptive threat response, i.e. pain. And it is clear that some people "maintain balances" (rolling debt) in their life due to work and family stress, sleep behaviors, exercise (or lack thereof) and physical movements (often compromised in some way), previous injuries or traumas, nutrition, gut microbiome, and so forth.

Given this understanding, approaches that just "mask the pain" or that the brain may perceive as increased risk (e.g. movements or therapies which the brain interprets as increased threat) versus putting the person in a position in which they can reduce their "threat debt" may in time make the person worse off. Approaches that help a little are a bit like making minimum payments: the person hasn't hit their limit, they seem asymptomatic, but they're just a single event away from being pushed over that limit. And using drugs to dull the pain may have the same impact as dulling the reality of our credit card debt with alcohol. It makes us feel better in the moment, but it doesn't necessarily change the circumstances that led to that debt, and in fact could be making us worse.

We'll explain in more detail how Scrambler Therapy works a bit later, but essentially, it facilitates a process which allows the brain to change and break up the neurotags, or neuroconnections associated to the Threat Neuromatrix, by giving the brain new information. We look at ST as a vital way to reduce the "threat debt" and to do it in a way that, for many, is akin to making substantial payments against that debt. Now, back to Dave.

CHRONIC PAIN EPIDEMIOLOGY AND TREATMENT OPTIONS

The incidence of chronic pain in the general population is staggering. According to the Institute of Medicine, approximately 100 million Americans suffer from chronic pain at an annual cost of between $560 billion and $635 billion (yes, that is *billion*), and for a significant number of these individuals, pain control is inadequate.[7] This is greater than the number of Americans that suffer from diabetes, heart disease, stroke, and cancer combined.[8] According to the Global Industry Analysts Report, between 3 and 4.5 percent of the world's population suffers from chronic neuropathic pain (a subtype of chronic pain that Scrambler Therapy is particularly successful at treating) for a total of between 222 and 333 million individuals across the globe with chronic neuropathic pain. This rate increases with age, and so the aging population will just cause these numbers to increase significantly.[9]

One of the reasons Global Industry Analysts has evaluated this industry is because of the universally discouraging results of current treatment options. Even a casual analysis of the satisfaction of chronic pain patients with the

7   Institute of Medicine, *Relieving Pain in America: A Blueprint for Transforming Prevention, Care, Education, and Research* (Washington, DC: Institute of Medicine, 2011)

8   American Academy of Pain Medicine, "AAPM Facts and Figures on Pain," http://www.painmed.org/patientcenter/facts_on_pain.aspx#refer

9   Global Industry Analysts, Inc. Report (January 10, 2011).

adequacy of their treatment regimens shows that it ranges close to the approval rating of the US Congress.[10] Chronic pain is a huge problem for primary care physicians for these same reasons.[11] As a primary care physician that has been in clinical practice for thirty years, I can say that the adequacy of our current tools to treat chronic pain is woeful. It is very difficult to see patients that you have known for years or decades continue to suffer despite trying multiple treatment modalities with little result. Telling a patient there is really nothing more you can do for them is frustrating and unrewarding.

Current treatment options for chronic pain can be divided into five main categories: medications, physical modalities, electrical modalities, procedures, and alternative medicine.

MEDICATIONS

These primarily fall into three main categories: opioids, neuroleptics, and antidepressants.

Opioids: Medicines such as oxycodone, Dilaudid, and fentanyl are hardly worth mentioning, as the problems

---

10 David Michaelson & Company, LLC, "Voices of Chronic Pain, A National Study," Conducted for American Pain Foundation.

11 Carole C. Upshur, Roger S. Luckmann, and Judith A. Savageau, "Primary Care Provider Concerns about Management of Chronic Pain in Community Clinic Populations," *Journal of General Internal Medicine* 21, no. 6 (2006): 652–655.

associated with them are so widely recognized that a discussion on them is not worth the paper upon which this report is printed.

Neuroleptics: This category primarily includes medications that were originally developed to treat seizure disorders, such as gabapentin (Neurontin), pregabalin (Lyrica), topiramate (Topamax), carbamazepine (Tegretol), lamotrigine (Lamictal), etc. There are three main problems with these medications. First, they all have significant side-effect profiles. Second, they can be very challenging to wean off of when discontinuing. And finally, they have never been shown[12] to be very effective for chronic pain.[13]

Antidepressants: There are many antidepressants on the market, old and new. All have been used to try to treat chronic pain, but there is no consensus that they work. The medication that has probably been studied the most is duloxetine (Cymbalta), but a Cochrane review found little evidence to support its effectiveness, and it has a significant incidence of side effects.[14]

---

12 National Institute for Health and Care Excellence, "Neuropathic Pain in Adults: The Pharmacological Management of Neuropathic Pain in Adults in Non-specialist Settings," NICE Clinical Guideline No. 173 (2013).

13 R. D. Rao et al., "Efficacy of Gabapentin in the Management of Chemotherapy-induced Peripheral Neuropathy," *Cancer* 110, no. 9 (2007): 2110–2118.

14 M. P. Lunn, R. A. Hughes, and P. J. Wiffen, "Duloxetine for Treating Painful Neuropathy, Chronic Pain or Fibromyalgia" Cochrane Database of Systematic Reviews CD007115 (2014).

PHYSICAL MODALITIES

Passive therapy such as massage therapy, ultrasound, traction, and iontophoresis are frequently advocated and used for chronic pain. All of these therapies have been shown to potentially provide short-term relief, but none have been shown to have any long-term impact on chronic pain syndromes.[15] Physical therapy and chiropractic and osteopathic manipulation are also common treatment forms, but most studies do not show any lasting benefits above and beyond placebo.[16]

ELECTRICAL MODALITIES

The two primary forms of electrical treatments for chronic pain are transcutaneous electrical nerve stimulation (TENS) and implantable nerve stimulators.

TENS: When people first learn of Scrambler Therapy, they often confuse it with TENS; however, they are completely different (this will be explained in more detail later). TENS is designed to "override" the pain signal by stimulating the A-delta nerve fiber and suppressing the perception of pain. It is not designed for long-term relief, as it only provides relief while the device is attached.

---

15 American Chronic Pain Association, *ACPA Resource Guide to Chronic Pain Medication & Treatment* (Rocklin, CA: ACPA, 2015), 115.

16 J. S. Feine and J. P. Lund, "An Assessment of the Efficacy of Physical Therapy and Physical Modalities for the Control of Chronic Musculoskeletal Pain," *Pain* 71, no. 1 (1997): 5-23.

There is little to no evidence that TENS is beneficial in chronic pain.[17] Recently, several companies have come out with wearable TENS devices, which can be worn on a more frequent basis, but again doing little to actually resolve the pain long-term.

Implantable nerve stimulators: Implantable nerve stimulators come in two forms, peripheral nerve stimulators (PNS) and spinal cord stimulators (SCS). Both are surgically implanted with electrodes, similar to a pacemaker, in order to provide continuous stimulation of the targeted nerve. In a sense, it is like a TENS unit that is implanted so it can be used long-term. A systematic review of the studies on spinal cord stimulators concluded that there is an "urgent need for randomized, controlled, long-term studies" with larger patient sample sizes.[18]

PROCEDURES

Invasive procedures include epidural steroid injections, nerve ablation procedures, and surgery.

Epidural steroid injections: This common procedure is performed by inserting a needle just outside the spinal sac and injecting a corticosteroid around the spinal nerve as

---

17   The Cochrane Collaboration and published in The Cochrane Library 2014, Issue 7

18   T. Cameron, "Safety and Efficacy of Spinal Cord Stimulation for the Treatment of Chronic Pain: A 20-year Literature Review," *Journal of Neurosurgery* 100, Spine 3 (2004): 254-267.

it exits the spinal foramina or into the facet joint, depending on what the physician is trying to accomplish. This is typically done under radiographic imaging guidance, but is still sometimes performed blindly. Despite the fact that there are over 9 million epidural steroid injections performed each year in the US, at an average cost of just under $2,000 per procedure,[19] there is very little evidence of long-term relief from chronic pain.[20] In fact, the medical literature is now suggesting that steroid injections actually accelerate the degeneration of tissue. Short-term gains at a long-term cost.

This was underscored for me when I attended a medical conference in London on October 13, 2015, sponsored by the Royal Society of Medicine, titled, "Chronic Pain and Psychiatry: Hype, Hope, and Facts." The conference was co-sponsored by the pain management and psychiatry sections of the Royal Society. The basic theme of the conference seemed to be something like, "Since we don't have any adequate treatments for chronic pain, we need our psychiatry colleagues to help chronic pain patients cope with their conditions." In fact, the section on epidural steroid injections was presented by Dr. Rajesh Munglani, Honorary Consultant in Pain Medicine for the National

---

19 Pat Anson, "Experts Say Epidural Steroid Injections Overused," *Pain News Network*, August 19, 2015.

20 S. Abdi et al., "Epidural Steroids in the Management of Chronic Spinal Pain: A Systematic Review," *Pain Physician* 10, no. 1 (2007): 185-212.

Health Service Trust. After admitting that there was no solid research data to support the benefits of epidural steroid injections, he expressed that it was still his belief that they do help some people.

Nerve ablation procedures: Often referred to as radiofrequency nerve ablation or radiofrequency neurotomy, this procedure involves using energy in the radiofrequency range to cause necrosis (destruction) of the targeted nerve fibers, with the intent of eliminating the source of the pain. Ablation treatment is often performed in patients that get only temporary relief from epidural steroid injections and is becoming increasingly popular, at a typical cost of $5,000. Multiple treatments are not uncommon.[21] Again, the problem is that there is no strong evidence that the treatment is effective.[22]

Surgery: Although there are many different types of surgeries done for pain, various forms of spine surgery are by far the most common surgeries done for chronic pain. Costs for such surgery, including hospitalization, anesthesia, rehab, etc., usually runs into the tens of thousands and occasionally hundreds of thousands of dollars. There is a

---

21 "Radiofrequency Neurotomy Insurance Claims and Lawsuits," Minnesota Injury Law (2009), http://minnesotaaccidentlawyer.blogspot.com/2009/02/radiofrequency-neurotomy-insurance.html

22 Stasia Bochnowski Muhlner, "Review Article: Radiofrequency Neurotomy for the Treatment of Sacroiliac Joint Syndrome," *Current Reviews in Musculoskeletal Medicine* 2, no. 1 (2009): 10–14.

lot of controversy about spine procedures, but one thing is obvious: a very high percentage of patients do not get significant resolution of their pain. A review done by the Rothman Institute showed that, in 2002, over 1 million spinal procedures were done in the US, and the lifetime prevalence of failed back surgery syndrome (FBSS) is 60 to 85 percent.[23] Those are pretty daunting statistics. It is common practice amongst primary care doctors to try to do anything you can to help your patients avoid spine surgery and only perform surgery as a last resort. Yet look how common it is, despite our efforts. When I was in medical school on the surgery rotation I learned the surgeon's motto: "A chance to cut is a chance to cure." If only they had filled in the statistics of what those chances actually were!

COMPLEMENTARY AND ALTERNATIVE MEDICINE (CAM)

A detailed review of the myriad of CAM options, including acupuncture, for the treatment of chronic pain is beyond the scope of this discussion, though Brendon has touched on many of them. The National Institutes of Health sponsor a division called the National Center for Complementary and Integrative Health. According to the information from the division's report on chronic pain, "The currently available evidence is not strong enough to

---

23   Rothman Institute, "Failed Back Spine Surgery," (2014), http://aocpmr.org/wp-content/uploads/2014/04/Failed-back-surgery-syndrome.pdf

allow definite conclusions to be reached about whether any complementary approach is effective for chronic pain."[24]

OVERVIEW OF SCRAMBLER THERAPY

Professor Giuseppe Marineo at the Center for Medical Research and Bioengineering at the University of Rome is the inventor of Scrambler Therapy. A biophysicist, Professor Marineo's initial research was on tissue regeneration, particularly liver regeneration. Later, medical colleagues who were aware of his work introduced him to Rita Levi-Montalcini, credited with discovering nerve growth factor, and she convinced him to join the emerging area of nerve regeneration. It was during this phase of his career that he became an expert in neuroanatomy and physiology. It was also during this time that he became aware of the extreme suffering that so many patients with chronic neuropathic pain were having to endure, with no significantly successful treatment remedies available. It was as he looked more closely at this problem that he came to understand that while the Gate Control Theory of pain did quite well in explaining acute pain, it was wholly inadequate in explaining chronic pain in general, and chronic neuropathic pain in particular. As he turned his research

---

24 National Center for Complementary and Integrative Health, "Chronic Pain: In Depth," NCCIH Pub No.: D456, last modified August 2015, https://nccih.nih.gov/health/pain/chronic.htm

efforts to this area, he developed the Information Theory of chronic pain, and his Scrambler Therapy device was developed based on the principles of this theory.

Although never officially labeled thus by Professor Marineo, the Information Theory of chronic pain, as we call it, takes into account the fact that the action potentials (nerve signals) sent by peripheral nerves to the brain are not just monotonous electrical signals, but are actually information-laden. In Marineo's own words:

> Letters assembled in a random manner, although recognizable as signals, do not constitute information. Similarly, action potentials generated sequentially by a stimulated receptor cannot be interpretable without an analytical model of "information coding" rules. For example, frequency modulation of action potentials gives us an idea of the stimulus intensity, but it does not tell us how its perception is coded in terms of different sensations, nor does it tell us how thermal sensation is coded differently from painful sensation with respect to information. Actually, based on simple coding of information in frequency modulation, it would theoretically and technically be possible to artificially reproduce any kind of sensation, but we know this is not so. This problem of coding/decoding system analysis in the central nervous system (CNS) does not limit itself only to frequency modulation. If

this were true, any type of sensory trick could have achieved it using very simple technologies.

Marineo continues:

> During the development of Scrambler Therapy, artificial neurons were developed to transmit to the CNS information recognizable as "self" and "non-pain" in a non-invasive manner through surface C receptors. Compared to the conventional electro-analgesia, the assumed active principle that is currently under trial is not to inhibit pain transmission (through A-beta fiber excitation), but to substitute pain information with synthetic "non-pain" information.[25]

This information is not only sent to the brain for processing, but in the case of chronic pain in particular, is manipulated by the brain in numerous ways, including the more complex cortical functions of memory and learning. This complex treatment by the brain of these electrical action potentials is what results in both the extreme variation of pain interpretation from individual to individual as well as the brain's ability to relearn how to deal with these action potentials.

The brain's ability to reestablish new neurological

---

25 "Scrambler Therapy Theory Bases," Delta Research & Development, accessed June 20, 2018. http://www.scramblertherapy.org/scrambler-therapy-theory-bases.htm

pathways to deal with errant messages is known as neuroplasticity and has been shown to be quite remarkable in many aspects.[26] An example that I think everyone can relate to is the unfortunate individual who has suffered a stroke. In the majority of cases, the most profound deficits that the individual experiences are immediately after the stroke, and it is very common for these individuals to regain a significant amount of their lost functionality (in some cases all of it) over time. This regaining of function does not occur because the brain replaces the dead neurons or grows new ones, although this may play some role. Rather, the improved function occurs primarily because of the brain's ability to "rewire," so to speak, different pathways that utilize healthy brain cells to accomplish the functions that had been lost. This ability of the brain to relearn function is a classic example of neuroplasticity. Neuroimaging studies have shown how areas of the brain that normally perform a completely different function are able to adapt and "take over" the performance of these functions that were lost due to the stroke.

Professor Marineo theorized that if the brain can do such marvelous things with motor function, why not with chronic pain? After years of research, Marineo was able to recreate action potentials that were consistent with

---

26   Eberhard Fuchs and Gabriele Flügge, "Review Article: Adult Neuroplasticity: More Than 40 Years of Research," *Neural Plasticity* 2014 (2014).

normal "non-pain" signals that are generated by healthy neurons that are not under duress.

Acute pain is primarily transmitted by larger, fast-signaling myelinated nerve fibers, primarily A-beta and A-delta fibers. In contrast to acute pain, chronic pain signals are primarily carried on thinner, unmyelinated nerves known as C-fibers. In a sense, Scrambler Therapy acts like an artificial neuron that utilizes healthy surface C-fibers surrounding the damaged nerves to send the "non-pain" signals to the brain for processing. This is done by placing surface electrodes (similar to ECG leads) just outside of the area of the patient's pain. With proper lead placement, the brain will accept these "non-pain" signals as normal and eventually replace the pain signals with them. This process results in almost immediate relief of the pain. The electrodes are then left in place for thirty to forty-five minutes as the Scrambler Therapy device sends cycles of variations of the "non-pain" signals up the healthy nerves to the brain. Although pain relief is almost immediate, in order to attain long-term relief, the process needs to utilize the neuroplasticity of the brain and several (typically about ten to twenty) consecutive daily treatments are required to accomplish this and give durability to the pain relief. Long-term can mean anything from thirty days to indefinitely. For those who get a recurrence of their pain, occasional "booster" treatments are needed to maintain perpetual pain relief.

When individuals first hear of Scrambler Therapy, it is not uncommon for them to confuse it with TENS devices or neurostimulators. However, the difference is fundamental. Both TENS and implantable neurostimulators are designed to override pain signals on the affected nerves. Neither is designed to retrain the brain in regard to pain perception, so there is no significant long-term effect from either device unless they are actively functioning. Scrambler Therapy, on the other hand, is designed to use neuroplasticity to retrain the brain to accept a "non-pain" signal in place of the pain signal and thus gives both more complete and longer lasting relief.

Although Scrambler Therapy was specifically developed for chronic neuropathic pain, experience has shown that it is effective for nearly all types of chronic pain. Below is a list of different types of pain that have been successfully treated by Scrambler Therapy at Radiant Pain Relief Centres:

- Abdominal pain
- Brachial plexus neuropathy
- Cancer pain
- Cervical neck pain
- Chemo-induced peripheral neuropathy (CIPN)
- Complex regional pain syndrome (CRPS)
- Degenerative disc disease
- Degenerative joint disease

- Diabetic neuropathy
- Failed back surgery syndrome
- Herniated discs
- HIV neuropathy
- Low back pain
- Lumbar radiculopathy
- Nerve entrapment (pinched) pain
- Nerve root compression
- Neuropathic pain
- Pelvic pain
- Phantom limb pain
- Postherpetic neuralgia (PHN or shingles)
- Postsurgical neuropathic pain
- Pudendal neuralgia
- Regional headache pain
- Sciatica
- Spinal stenosis
- Trigeminal neuralgia
- Vulvodynia
- Whiplash

SUCCESS STORIES

The following are just a few patient success stories, with many more on our website and Facebook page. I recognize that these few and even the hundreds of others that we have collectively amassed since beginning February 2014 are "statistically insignificant" as it relates to scientific proof. But for these patients it is not insignificant. It is life changing. I share a few stories for illustration purposes of the types of outcomes we see. Many more testimonials can be found on our website.

CASE #1: TOM K.—CIPN

Tom K. is a thirty-nine-year-old male survivor of a germ cell tumor who had over six years of severe chemotherapy-induced peripheral neuropathy (CIPN) in his feet that prevented him from sleeping and participating in his hobbies, and dramatically impacted his career as an attorney. He was only able to wear specialized shoes, and only for short periods of time, and was unable to travel. At his demo, his starting pain was 7/10 and ended at 0/10. His schedule prevented him from having consecutive treatments as we recommend, but he ended up with durable pain relief after seventeen treatments. Three months later, his pain started to return, so he had a booster and a series of three boosters one month later. He has remained pain-free since, and is able to wear normal shoes, travel, and even hike again, despite not being on any pain medications.

CASE #2: LANA R.—PHN

Lana R. is a fifty-four-year-old female who presented with severe postherpetic neuralgia (PHN) on her trunk, from which she had been suffering for ten years. She was on disability, and had previously been working as a sheriff. As is typical, over that ten years, she had tried every treatment she could find, but without success. She had her initial demo, and even five days later, her presenting pain for her first treatment had dropped from 8/10 to 6/10, and again she left at a 0/10. After her sixth treatment, she had twelve days of complete pain relief. When it returned a few weeks later, she had three booster sessions, and her pain was gone for eight days. A single booster a few days later gave her sixteen days of relief. Her last booster was many months ago, she remains pain-free, and she says that she has her life back. She plays with her grandkids and is actively looking for a job, and Radiant has helped another patient get off disability.

CASE #3: GREG B.—FBSS

Greg B. is a fifty-three-year-old male who had fifteen months of chronic pain from failed back surgery syndrome (FBSS). His pain was preventing him from driving as well as participating in all the exercise that he enjoyed, such as racquetball, tennis, and golf. When he presented for the last of his initial treatments, his pain area had decreased from large areas on his low back, anterior leg, and posterior leg to just a small residual area on his low back. He presented for that last treatment of his initial series at only a 3/10 and was zeroed out with that treatment. After three weeks, his pain started to return a bit, and he came in for a single booster and got his pain down to 0/10 and has been well ever since. Greg says that he is back to all of his normal activities. He enjoys racquetball, tennis, and golf once more. He is thrilled with the freedom of being able to drive again.

CASE #4: PAM S.—TGN

Pam S. is a fifty-nine-year-old female who has been a patient of mine for over twenty years. She had been suffering for eight years with severe chronic pain due to trigeminal neuralgia (TGN). I had referred her to multiple doctors, and she tried numerous treatments, including multiple meds, naturopathy, and acupuncture, all without benefit. Just the wind on her face was unbearable, so this very outdoorsy woman had become isolated. She stopped traveling, stopped working, and was essentially homebound. She presented for her demo treatment at an 8/10 and left at 0/10. After her initial treatment series, she required a few intermittent boosters, but has had minimal to no pain for over two years now. Pam is ecstatic about having her life back. She travels to visit her grandkids; she goes outside in all sorts of inclement weather, and basically lives a normal life. All of this she thought would be impossible just two years ago, before she started treatment.

THE NEAR DEATH OF A NOVEL TECHNOLOGY

As we evaluate and understand the context of the current thinking about chronic pain, the fragmentation of the care providers addressing chronic pain, the drivers and limitations of those treatments, and the dramatic shift in pain science understanding from what most clinicians have been trained on and from which they currently get paid, we can better understand the reality of why an innovative solution like ST has had difficulty taking root. Categorically and fundamentally, ST is novel—novel in its underlying theory, novel in its mechanism of action, and certainly novel in its results. Dave has provided a fairly easy to understand description of this technology and its origins. "Too good to be true," some might say. And "too good to be true" is more easily dismissed than it is adopted, particularly if it challenges the status quo thinking and may impact the economics of that status quo.

When Dave and I ordered our first ST device and opened our first pilot clinic in February 2014, we did not intend to try to seek exclusivity for the technology; we thought we might have the basis for a better business model, but our priority was really first around three things:

1. To prove the technology actually worked as well as we hoped it did. Since then, we have learned so much and actually believe that it is better than the studies and other outcome stories previously illustrated. But

we know with equal certainty that it has to be done the right way—there are clearly more effective ways of treating patients and consistency in outcomes that are born solely from understanding, learning, and following the right protocols of care and delivery.

2. To figure out a pricing model that would make therapy affordable despite a lack of insurance coverage, and still allow us to build a viable company. This was a learning process, but we have done this in a creative way, which could not likely be replicated in any other care environment. Therapy is affordable and accessible, and the company has a sustainable revenue model.

3. To see if we could create a foundation upon which we could eventually scale the solution more broadly. After years of clinical practice and many hundreds of patients treated in our pilot operations, we have done the work, put in the time, and learned by doing it, giving us confidence and knowledge about what works and what doesn't. Our business solution, though equally novel to the innovative device we use, creates a strong foundation for scale and growth. Later, I will make the case for why I believe that this is the best, most viable model for scale and expansion—at least initially.

By the time I approached Dave about ST in the summer of 2013, I had already concluded that a different business model was necessary to effectively commercialize the technology. After a few years of limited success, but seeing some firsthand outcomes that were nothing short of impressive and hearing the results that other demos, clinical studies, and the handful of clinicians using ST were achieving, I began to think the issue of commercialization was not product viability, but in this case, the model being commercialized. This got me thinking and exploring the obstacles, and whether or not a solution could be built to overcome or mitigate those obstacles.

As I analyzed it, the following facts emerged as the dominant barriers to commercialization. Some are organic; some were created by or made worse through the former licensee's approach and limitations. But all, ultimately, were overcome by Radiant's business model.

FDA-510(k): When the former licensee took ST through the FDA clearance process, in an effort to save time and money, they predicated this novel, categorically different, and innovative therapy on TENS therapy, actually calling it "Scrambler Therapy MC-5A TENS Device." TENS, as discussed briefly by Dave previously, is transcutaneous electrical nerve stimulation technology, which has been around for fifty or more years. TENS works on the Gate Control Theory of chronic pain, can provide some analgesic benefits short-term, but does little to resolve chronic pain or provide lasting relief. This is underscored by the several companies that are now marketing wearable TENS units, allowing the relief to become more mobile, but illustrating that it must be on and applied to provide benefits.

This TENS classification has, in part, limited the medical establishment's inclination to investigate or understand ST's novel mechanism of action and superior results. Furthermore, Medicare, which typically sets the rate at which treatments would be reimbursed (i.e. what insurance companies will pay for a particular procedure), based its initial recommendation on the rate of TENS therapy—something in the ballpark of thirty-five dollars per treatment session. The Current Procedural Terminology or CPT code that was assigned to the therapy was considered an exploratory code. These two factors make a viable insurance reimbursement model unlikely and unsustainable, particularly when we evaluate the aspects of the economics surrounding delivery of ST inside a clinic.

Economics and costs of delivery: The retail price, or the price that a clinician would pay for an ST device, fluctuated in the years I was associated with the former licensee and trying to sell the equipment. When I began marketing the technology, the retail price we "sold" a device for was around $80,000. The price increased over the years, though, as I mentioned previously, some of the earliest "buyers" paid substantially less than that, or received their equipment at no cost.

In a move akin to the thinking of Martin Shkreli, aka "Pharma Boy"—the novice pharmaceutical company CEO who raised prices on his critical drug from $13.50 a pill to $750 a pill because people needed it, there was no other strong competitor to it, and he felt that the necessity of demand would support it—the former licensee decided that, due to the novelty of ST, a retail above $100,000 per device was justified. Maybe it would have been if there had been demand for it, understanding about it, and viable revenue potential for it, but this really only further stymied sales. A retail price in the six figures and no viable insurance reimbursement is a difficult combination of factors, particularly when thrown into the context of other economic, operating, and institutional-thinking factors outlined previously. For a clinician to justify a fairly high-ticket price to buy a device, and to make money with ST, they'd have to be very comfortable with cash-model businesses, selling, marketing, and overcoming objections. Not only do physicians generally not have the time to do this, they typically lack both the appetite and the skillset to do it.

Physicians' training, perspectives, and biases: As discussed, physicians being trained primarily in biochemistry receive most of their formal education in understanding drugs and the mechanism of action of drugs in the body. They are not typically trained in biophysics—so a biophysical therapy approach like that of ST is not immediately fully understood, particularly without also understanding the latest pain science. Therefore, it becomes much easier to dismiss it as "snake oil" or to wait and see how the technology evolves.

As discussed earlier, physicians often develop rigidity in their thinking. Few are entrepreneurial. Few are sales and marketing oriented. And few are true early adopters, choosing (usually out of a genuine desire to protect their patients) to be rather conservative in their thinking towards and prescribing of new therapies. If they happen to be any of these things, the healthcare system, operating environment, and institutional rigidity—which all influence how they practice—make it very difficult to act in that manner. The combination of a costly piece of equipment that physicians aren't trained to understand, a therapy that sounds too good to be true, and an economic model that makes little sense, make ST a difficult technology to market in the traditional ways.

Of course, these are generalities; there are many types of clinicians and doctors, for some of whom this would be a sensible addition, and there have been a handful of enterprising clinicians who did purchase ST, one or two of who have created seemingly compelling business solutions. However, their clinical approach was nothing unique, not particularly patient-centered, not particularly novel nor scalable, and often key-man dependent (meaning that the doctor was heavily involved). I would argue that their status quo thinking and their own clinical biases, in the end, do little to advance ST as a scalable solution to the significant problem of chronic pain. By and large, they tried to make ST work within the confines of their existing clinical model and thinking: the MDs using ST would bill insurance for related procedures, office visits, anything they could, and try to charge out-of-pocket for the ST therapy (perhaps discounted) or try to bill insurance under some generic procedure code.

The chiropractors using it use it in conjunction with their other therapies and gadgets. Each clinician creates a different patient experience, price discrepancies, and a range of variable clinical outcomes. Ultimately, this variability becomes problematic in trying to illustrate to skeptical physicians, scientists, and consumers that ST has the potential to be a genuinely effective and reliable solution to the problem of chronic pain.

Getting my head around these facts lead me to new thinking about how to overcome these obstacles, and again context and history play a role. Having had the varied professional experience I have, I could see the landscape of healthcare. I knew the fragmentation of care and differences in methodology, approaches, and economic drivers, and I knew that because no one camp owns chronic pain, that no one camp could effectively own this novel therapy without some compromise. I also realized the limitations posed for each of these clinician types.

For most MDs/DOs (biomedical care), the economics and the patient throughput demand in either private practice/clinical practice settings or hospitals are difficult to overcome—and the understanding of, and the clinical evidence for ST don't justify the effort involved. Chiropractors remain the most likely candidates for acquiring and using ST, but focusing on them, or any of the other "complementary and alternative care" providers, most of whom have limited prescribing power, would further limit the appetite for and interest in, as well as reduce any chance of viable insurance coverage/mainstream adoption of, ST. It would forever cement it as "fringe" medicine in the minds of the medical establishment.

My argument and belief, upon identifying all of this, was that in order for ST to take off, it either needed a much stronger economic structure, supported by a deeper body of clinical evidence so that the medical establishment could really get behind it, or it needed such strong consumer demand that it would drive a shift in thinking amongst the medical establishment. Both of these options are very costly and time consuming, but it seemed to me that cultivating consumer interest was by far the more controllable one.

From my perspective, based upon conversations with

numerous doctors about ST's clinical evidence, there seemed to be a "damned if you do, damned if you don't" bias around it. The current body of evidence was too limited to be sufficient. But due to their training, perspective, and mindset about historical approaches for pain management that they perceive as "snake oil," even the most well-executed blinded studies with longitudinal outcomes, published in peer-reviewed journals, would be looked at suspiciously and skeptically—like the books were somehow "cooked." It seemed unlikely that the medical establishment would be early adopters of ST in any sort of significant fashion; there were just too many factors stacked against that reality. From this point forward, the thinking migrated from trying to make it work for the clinician to trying to make it work for the consumer.

Up until the early 1970s, it was illegal, and considered unethical, for healthcare companies to advertise. As this changed, and as healthcare institutions and later pharmaceutical companies could start to legally market, we saw how powerfully the consumer voice and opinion could shape the economics and delivery of healthcare. Having spent time professionally with hundreds of physicians and healthcare administrators, I have heard countless stories, both good and bad, about patients presenting with a demand for a certain drug or therapy because they saw an ad for it. This type of thinking, combined with the access to information and social networking, makes it almost impossible to overestimate the role consumers play in shaping healthcare today.

My belief about ST was that the consumers could be the voice and driving force for change, understanding and adopting the potential faster and at less cost than investing in research. And frankly, going direct to consumer is easier than trying to expand the institutional understanding that is spinning its wheels in antiquated treatments. The path to winning the hearts and minds of healthcare practitioners would be slower and less able to be controlled, and would require more research. Both a consumer approach and an institutional approach would have a cost, but it seemed that the cost of investment towards a direct-to-consumer approach would have the most certain and quickest potential for return, as well as begin to fill the dire need for effective chronic pain treatment.

And so the focus shifted away from a selling model and towards the consumer.

CHAPTER 4

A VISION AND MODEL FOR DISRUPTION

———

All truth passes through three stages. First, it is ridiculed. Second, it is violently opposed. Third, it is accepted as being self-evident.

—ARTHUR SCHOPENHAUER

This chapter discusses the previous experience and learning I had, specifically in the hearing aid industry, which allowed me to see and design a new model delivery of the technology.

I recently listened to a talk by Dr. Joe Dispenza in which he said something to the effect of "When you're trying to create something new, you'll always be considered a fool or insane because no one else is doing what you're doing.

It's unconventional. It's outside of the beliefs of a culture. But, if you pull it off, you'll be considered a genius."

I am not sure I will ever be considered a genius, but I can understand this quote and the intent behind it. Doing something new is lonely and isolating. In this chapter and the next, I'll share the thinking that went into modeling our business as a direct-to-consumer company and some of the obstacles and resistance we faced in that pursuit. It starts with the sexy topic of hearing aids.

A MODEL FOR SUCCESS

Hearing aids are generally not covered by insurance. And they are not particularly cheap. An average sales price for a set of hearing aids is around $6,000. Having spent years in the hearing aid industry, working with private practice audiologists and ear, nose, and throat physicians, I knew the drivers of success in profitable hearing aid clinics. I knew the methodologies of marketing, of selling an out-of-pocket solution, and of creating value and overcoming objections to drive sales, and I knew the nuance of doing that in a healthcare environment where neither the patient wants to be sold to, nor, generally speaking, does the practitioner want to be perceived as a salesperson. In this type of scenario, it comes down to two things:

1. The patient acknowledging a problem, so that the clinician can become a solution provider to that problem

2. The solution provider providing enough value in the solution to justify the cost of the investment on the part of the patient

All care has a cost, and if the value of that care is sufficient to justify the expense, then investment in the care is sensible—whether insurance covers all of it, part of it, or none of it. A cosmetic procedure purely for appearances may be hard to justify for some people, but if that procedure is to restore anatomy or normalcy following an accident or a disease, it might be more justifiable. It comes down to value. Indeed, for many individuals the discomfort, disruption, and discouragement that chronic pain imposes justify an investment in a better solution. And it seemed that we had a better value to offer than most other therapies available.

As I thought more deeply and analyzed the successful hearing aid center model as a template, I realized in that structure we had a very sensible model for clinical operations, scale, and growth. If people are willing to pay several thousand dollars out of pocket to resolve or improve their hearing loss, they're willing to pay something out of pocket to get out of chronic pain; it is just a matter of making them aware of it and having it presented to them the right way. So, the foundation, vision, and initial thinking for what would become Radiant Pain Relief Centres was born.

Similarities between a successful hearing aid center and a potential new-model pain clinic dedicated to this therapy include:

Similar cost structure: The initial capital outlay, or cost, to build and operate a hearing aid clinic is similar to what would be expected in our center. They include initial expenditure in equipment, tenant improvements, prelaunch marketing, and cash to cover ongoing operations as revenues build. The ongoing operating expenses are fairly stable and predictable: rent, utilities, payroll and related, and marketing. While there are some differences in the ongoing operating costs, they were close enough to give us a starting point in building a budget.

Similar revenue potential (and a suggested target for an average sales price): Knowing the topline revenue potential of a successful hearing aid center and the average sales price per hearing aid sold gives us both a revenue target potential and a basis for an estimate of what we would need to charge in order to build a viable company when replacing hearing care with ST therapy. As I modeled this initially, and later remodeled it with the help of brighter financial minds, we arrived at an estimated average price that we would need to command in order to justify the business. Of course, we didn't know for sure if we were right or wrong, in terms of the market's response. Would they pay that rate? Only time would tell, but that gave us a basis to begin.

Similar marketing aspect: Given the out-of-pocket cost of hearing aids, and that of our therapy, there is a need to advertise more so than there is for most other healthcare practices. But more than just recognizing the need for advertising, building something new allowed us to think of marketing more completely, and to innovate the whole of the delivery around the Four Ps of Marketing:

- The **product** (what we offer and how we offer it)
- The **price** (how we price the product or service, the value behind it, and what pricing says about the product or service)
- The **place** (how the place feels, the experience it creates, accessibility, etc.)
- **Promotion** (how we advertise and promote the solution)

Marketing professors also taught me that a fifth P is sometimes an important marketing consideration. That fifth P is **people** and, given the personal and intimate service we provide, having the right people is something that also received a lot of consideration initially, and certainly ongoing, as we've been building. These are all serious considerations that translate into successful commercialization, and along with values, mission, and vision begin to form the basis of the business's brand. The hearing aid clinic model, as a consumer business with a retail component, provided a strong basis of experience and initial thought, but a lot of original thinking also went into the modeling of our center.

I wanted to create a patient experience and build a brand that was different from most other healthcare centers and clinical experiences. I wanted to exceed expectations beyond what people knew they might have. I wanted to build a disruptive consumer service brand.

Similar operating drivers, patient throughputs, and KPIs: The operating drivers (revenues versus costs), the volume and flow of patients, and the key performance indicators (KPIs) that reflect the vitality and progress of the business are certainly different in our center than in a successful hearing aid business. However, by understanding and modeling the other factors—costs, revenue targets, the marketing aspect, etc.—certain assumptions could be modeled fairly easily. By understanding the drivers of the business, things become measurable, predictable, and adjustable. Although some unique learning went in, and continues to go in as our business intelligence and data grow, the hearing aid clinic model provided a starting point of analysis and modeling.

Similar profit potential: With the cost and revenues modeled, all the aspects of marketing considered, and the operating drivers calculated, potential for profitability becomes clear—either it is a viable business model or it is not. As the model was built and refined, and the numerous variables massaged, it became clear that, on paper, this model could work very well. If the assumptions held in real life, if patients saw the value and invested in therapy at the estimated revenue amount we forecasted, we had a business that could be profitable, while still being rather affordable. But even if we were wrong, we had a plan, and the only way to prove a plan is to put it into action and test it.

Spending more time with this concept, working it out in my mind and on paper, I realized that this model would not only work to give a viable operating structure to a direct-to-consumer business built around this technology, but in fact it would overcome most, if not all, of the market obstacles and barriers outlined in the previous chapter.

A direct-to-consumer business meant that we could bypass the skeptical medical professional. The price of the technology and a lack of insurance coverage became less of an issue; if we could create the right value proposition and price point, patients would pay for it, justifying the investment in the technology. We could also likely negotiate a wholesale price for the devices based upon making multiple device purchases and pushing our price down. The lack of a deep and robust body of clinical studies became less of an issue because, generally speaking, the consumers don't care as much about placebo controls and peer-reviewed studies.

Consumers like knowing that the Mayo Clinic and Johns Hopkins University are the primary research centers—a true fact—and that the chief medical officer overseeing the training and care process is a Harvard/MIT-trained medical doctor with thirty years of clinical experience and a great reputation—also a true fact. But above all, they care whether or not it will be a better solution to their problem of chronic pain. They don't care about theoretics and statistics; they care about getting out of bed, about functioning, and about rekindling hope that pain does not control their life anymore. We believed we could offer them these things and more.

The FDA-510(k) allows us to market to patients that the technology was indeed FDA-cleared, a comforting and appealing aspect to any therapy, and one that helps it rise above the perception of "snake oil" to many consumers. The type of classification (class II) allowed us to not require a prescription or physician involvement in administering the therapy. In this case, the TENS classification is actually valuable to us. ST treatment is very safe.

Very clear contraindications (or disqualifiers) exist: pregnancy, implanted device, and certain medications. In all the years of research and use, there have been no reported side effects beyond some occasional mild skin irritation, tiredness during or following treatment, or rarely, a slight and temporary increase in pain (often followed by reduced pain, lower than baseline). This meant that we could go confidently to the consumer with a safe solution. The questions really became: Does it actually work, how quickly, and for how long, etc.? If it does work, could we figure out a pricing model that would be viable to the company and yet affordable to the average person despite a lack of insurance coverage? And lastly, could we build a foundation for growth?

It was this concept—of a new chronic pain treatment business, modeled after a successful hearing aid clinic, but built around ST—that I presented to Dave in the summer of 2013. After the treatment demo trials that were conducted on his patients later that year, we made plans to buy our first device and open a center. We ordered a device from the former licensee, and in February 2014, we opened our first center.

CHAPTER 5

THE SAFEST, MOST CONSISTENTLY EFFECTIVE AND APPEALING SOLUTION TO THE EPIDEMIC OF CHRONIC PAIN

———

Trust is built with consistency.

—LINCOLN CHAFEE

This chapter discusses the real-time learning and experience that helped evolved the Radiant business model.

As we began to operate with the Scrambler Therapy

technology in February 2014, we began to see results immediately and, while we were making some money from treatment revenues, we really looked at this as a learning opportunity. I joked then, and still do now, that our first little pilot center was the equivalent of our Hewlett-Packard garage. It ended up being a much deeper learning process than we/I had expected, but one I look back at now with gratitude and appreciation.

There is a big difference between theory and actuality, and there is no substitute for real-world learning as we began to put our business plan into action. In the following chapter, I'll discuss some of the many challenges we faced in building Radiant, but I can confidently say that there is real value when you're faced with opposition and you have to respond. It either makes you better, or it breaks you. I believe it has made us better, and that betterment has uniquely qualified us to deliver to the world this new approach. In this chapter, I'll talk through some of the factors and learning that we've gone through that have shaped our vision for our business model, and the delivery and evolution of this therapy.

As discussed before, chronic pain is very complicated. It is very individual, multifactorial, and often layered with complexity in the form of emotions and individual identification that gets tied to it. In our business model we are seeking to address this very complicated problem in a simple and elegant way. But it is also important to understand and recognize that the business, particularly for a new, disruptive business, is also complicated and multifactorial. Most businesses fail. They fail because there are many things that can go wrong, and even if everything goes right, success is not guaranteed. As discussed previously, there are a lot of drivers that prevent innovation and disruption in the whole of healthcare, so we chose to build our model outside of the traditional healthcare setting—without insurance, building centers to create a whole new experience, and hopefully a strong brand, capable of shifting people's understanding about pain and, of course, their access to our approach to it.

Very early on, we began seeing phenomenal patient outcomes and learning more each day; we had a growing confidence that we were onto something. Being that we devoted our full-time energy to using, understanding, and improving our delivery of the therapy (something no other clinic had done, as ST was simply an additional part-time therapy integrated into existing clinics), over time we became consistently quite good, but we knew we needed to keep learning more. We invested in sending several members of our staff, including Dr. Farley, our training nurse, and me, to Rome for training directly with the device inventor, Professor Giuseppe Marineo. This training, coupled with our own growing clinical intelligence and sophistication, helped us continue to refine our model and improve our clinical results even further. We were growing, improving every day, and optimistic in our plan and vision, with the clinical results exceeding our expectations and the business results showing real promise.

THE BIRTH OF OUR MISSION STATEMENT AND OUR BABY STEPS OF GROWTH

Indeed, we were becoming more sophisticated, more polished, professional, and confidently consistent in our clinical delivery, but also in our business processes. We felt that, without effective business delivery, the therapy could never really be grown in a significant way. So, we focused equally on the business modeling and delivery and on the clinical—again, I believe that we are the only clinic in the world to have done this. And our focus was not how to make it "fit into the healthcare model," but how to develop and deliver the *best* model to support this novel approach and create a platform for scale and expansion.

If we think about the most successful brands or businesses, no matter the industry, no matter the price point, no matter if it's a product or service business, the key and fundamental factor of success is one thing: consistency. Businesses that consistently deliver to their customers what their customers expect will likely succeed. Think about this: take Nordstrom and Walmart, two successful retail companies, though they are very different. The price points, the environments, the quality, the service, etc. are all different, but they are both highly successful. Why? Because they consistently deliver to their customer what their customer expects. The Walmart customer is not expecting a Nordstrom product, price point, or service level and vice versa. Businesses that fail to remember this, fail to stay around. History is full of businesses that lost sight of this fundamental concept of consistency in their business or in a certain product, and resulted in failure.

So, we've focused on processes, training, and systems to help ensure consistency in the clinical delivery of our therapy, as well as the business delivery. I spent many years building systems for consistency, improved outcomes, and patient results in healthcare settings, the hearing aid industry in particular, so I had good insight into where to begin. But in time, all of the systems mentioned benefited and were refined through real-world learning. They will continue to be refined because we've baked into our business systems a culture that is focused on continual improvement. It influences our hiring, our training, our expectations of each other, our communications, and our care and business delivery.

Over time, our process tightened and we refined it into something that we call PEP: Positive Experience Process. PEP became our methodology—how we answered the phone, communicated our value proposition, and described our therapy. PEP became our overarching methodology for consistent, optimized, patient-centered experience. I coached all the team in constructing an elevator pitch about what they/we did. We weren't a pain clinic, we weren't a medical clinic, and we weren't anything that had existed before.

We were changing the way chronic pain is understood and treated. We didn't have patients, or clients; we had members (most of our clients pay for treatment on an "annual membership"). This was new and exclusive. This became and remains our introductory statement. When asked, "What do you do?'" we answer, "I work for Radiant Pain Relief Centres; we're changing the way chronic pain is understood and treated." This leads to more interest: "What does that mean? Tell me more."

Our values became more than just words: Compassion, Honesty, Creativity, Ownership Spirit, and Doing the Right Thing—they became living things, tangible aspects of what we did every day in our pursuit of changing the way chronic pain is treated.

Around this time, a friend of mine told me a story about Phil Knight, the founder of Nike. In Oregon, Nike is the crown jewel of business and is studied and discussed a lot. Not long after Nike went public, they were really suffering.

Their stock price was falling. The market was challenging them. Reebok was dominating on a lower-priced, popular sneaker. Faced with some difficult decisions about how to respond, Knight disappeared into his office in contemplation, emerging some time later with a directive that would ultimately lead Nike to become the global sports apparel and footwear brand that it is: the best athletes, the best shoes, the best ads.

With all the things we do daily—answer the phone, greet clients, treat clients, clean and prepare treatment rooms, chart client notes, etc.—and with all things I, as CEO do—cultivate investors, deal with supply issues, attend meetings, etc.—I felt that I needed something to keep us focused on the things that matter the most. Something simple, yet powerful. Our operating mantra was born:

THE BEST TECHNOLOGY, THE BEST PEOPLE, THE BEST EXPERIENCE.

Indeed, we would change the way chronic pain is understood and treated, and we'd do it by identifying, utilizing, understanding, and ultimately evolving and developing the best technology. We'd do it by attracting, training and developing, and retaining the best people. And we'd do it by working collectively, collaboratively, and passionately to create the best experience—the best experience for each other as colleagues and, ultimately, the best experience for our clients. Our confidence in our ability to change our clients' lives for the better was matched only by our desire to do so, and to create the best possible experience for them each time they came to us. As a team, we were realizing that we had the safest, most consistently effective and appealing solution to this big problem of chronic pain and we were refining our expertise in delivering that solution.

Most medical clinics are not set up to accommodate this technology or this type of therapy. Beyond the high costs of equipment and a lack of viable insurance coverage, there are high opportunity costs that prevent most clinics from buying and implementing this technology. There is an opportunity cost of requiring a patient to sit for an hour while on this therapy treatment, for which they could command a relatively minimal amount of a few hundred an hour, compared to the throughput of patients through that same space in an hour and all their billable office visit and procedure charges, or the economics of a single injection therapy, which takes about fifteen minutes of physician time and earns the doctor $1,000 to $2,000. There is no comparison, and it is even more drastic when we understand that this is a process, not a procedure, meaning that the process of retraining the brain takes time. Some clients may need more initial treatments, some less. Some will need infrequent boosters, some more. It is an individual process that unfolds over time and requires a frequency of visits, initially and ongoing, which is different than what most existing clinics are set up to accommodate.

For new, innovative therapies to be successfully brought to market, there are many important factors which must be met to consider, such as the clinical environment, the technician, and the process. I briefly mentioned the Four Ps of Marketing earlier: product, price, place, and promotion. I want to spend a few minutes on each of these, to better understand the thinking that went into our model.

The first is the product, which is the therapy process, but it is also the experience that the client has in the center.

The second is the price: how it is priced helps frame the value of the treatment (e.g. Nordstrom prices versus Walmart prices).

The third is the place: how it looks, how it feels, where it is located, etc.

The fourth is the promotion: how it is advertised, what drives customer interest and behavior.

Though not traditionally part of the Four Ps of Marketing, "people" is sometimes considered a fifth P, and given the high-touch, personal experience involved in relieving someone's pain, we consider people to be an important component and consideration.

PRODUCT

The entirety of this book is primarily dedicated to better understanding our product, and the technology and methodology that underlie it. I don't need to spend a ton of time repeating it here. But to make the point, the product is "the safest, most consistently effective and appealing solution" to the epidemic of chronic pain. The product is a result of the outcome arrived at through novel technology and thoughtful delivery of that technology. The product and our delivery are enhanced by the consideration of all these aspects. We're fortunate to be able to think openly about each aspect and build a clinical and business solution to address the factors of success without the need to fit into an existing model and its incumbent obligations. To be able to think and build in a novel way allows us to really deliver a novel, disruptive solution.

It is also worth pointing out that the product is really a process, not a product as in a transactional good sold, and not even a procedure, like a surgical operation. The process of brain retraining is based upon the principle of neuroplasticity. Like anything the brain is learning, repetition and exposure are necessary to enact change, particularly lasting change. It becomes a process, not a procedure. Most medical clinics are set up for procedures. With our therapy, this typically means daily one-hour sessions for two to three weeks. For most patients, this type of consistency will result in significant, often total, relief that becomes lasting for an extended period of time. Periodic booster treatments are given to maintain results perpetually.

We've designed the Radiant Pain Relief Centres model to most effectively deliver care and support needed in the therapy process. There are no competing interests, no conflicts because one therapy is more lucrative than another or quicker to deliver. At the end of the day, we serve only one master, our client, with a focus on giving them the best care and result possible. This especially includes how we think about pricing, and the economic cascade that flows from the client's decision to purchase.

PRICE

I want to spend a bit of time talking through the pricing structure. I think this deserves some review of the thinking and learning that has gone into it, because at the end of the day the math has to work. If it doesn't, it does not matter how effective something is; if people can't afford it and companies and their shareholders can't make money, it's not very sustainable.

When we began, we had a pricing structure in place based upon what I had seen in the hearing aid industry and what we'd factored into our pricing models in the business plan. Underlying that pricing was a belief that "price is only an issue in the absence of value," meaning that value is really the determining factor.

"Value" is a relative term. For some, there is value in spending $200 on a shirt—because of its material, craftsmanship, style, fit, brand name, etc. To others, spending $200 on a shirt seems like a ridiculous thing, when a $19 shirt would do an equally fine job, covering the body and fulfilling its purpose. So, with that in mind, it is important to understand that no matter what we priced our therapy at, some people would say it's "too expensive," i.e. not valuable enough. And perhaps others would be so pleased to have their life back that they would literally be willing to pay anything.

It is unknown exactly how many treatments are going to be needed initially and what the frequency and quantity of boosters will be, so we look at it in snapshots of one year. This longer horizon of twelve months changes the perspective from both a therapy standpoint and a care delivery standpoint, which allows us to also change how we think about pricing. However, how we thought about pricing when we began has evolved substantially.

Knowing that we wanted to create a value proposition, and

recognizing that this therapy is a very different approach from the pain treatments that most of our clients had already experienced, from the first day we offered both a free initial "demo" session and package pricing. We gave all qualified clients (meaning that the client didn't have a disqualifying condition such as being pregnant or having an implanted medical device such as a pacemaker) a free demo treatment and presentation on the therapy, in which we explained the process of daily treatment sessions and periodic boosters. The pricing package we offered gave clients the option to pay for each session as they went, or to buy a package of ten sessions for a discount of 20 percent.

Seeing the value of the investment in therapy following the free demo, and the savings offered in the package, most clients bought the package. But having a package of ten sessions created its own unique challenges. Ten became a magic number. If optimal relief was achieved prior to ten, clients often wanted a refund on the unused sessions. If clients needed more, they would be disappointed because they had felt like the package of ten sessions implied that ten would fully resolve their pain, which was not always the case. They might be frustrated thinking about the need to buy more sessions à la carte or another package. And even if ten did resolve their pain, when the time came that their pain began to return and they needed a booster treatment session, often they would delay as long as possible, until it was absolutely necessary, instead of the advised "call us if your pain returns." By the time we saw them back it was like starting over. That's if we saw them back—many would consider that the therapy didn't really help because they now found themselves back in pain, forgot the profound relief that they had achieved, and would not return. This model didn't serve the client or the company.

We changed our thinking around price to better reflect that this is a process, and evolved pricing to be more like a gym membership, which gives clients access throughout the year. This membership model accomplishes at least two valuable things: 1) it makes treatment more affordable by spreading the cost out over time and 2) it encourages the appropriate level and necessary use of the process, which results in better outcomes and happier clients.

The annual membership model makes treatment at Radiant very affordable because the bulk of the cost of therapy is capped and spread out over the year, with a variable cost per treatment for heavier use that increases the price modestly and appropriately. While every patient may have a slightly different pattern of use and total number of sessions needed, a common number of treatments is around twenty sessions, with ten to fifteen sessions taking place in the first few weeks, and a few sets of boosters in the remaining eleven months. On the basic membership, the cost of this averages out to around ten dollars a day. For the cost of a couple of lattes each day, we can get and maintain relief—safely, consistently, and significantly.

Even though there is a cost, most clients tell us that it's the best investment they've made in the management of their pain. For many, it's a net neutral cost, as they redirect other costs each month for drug and therapy treatments that aren't working sufficiently and that have become unnecessary as they invest in Radiant's solution. Of course, the value they receive in getting their lives back and reclaiming themselves from the shackles of a life bound by chronic pain is, for many, priceless.

Pricing is very much part of the consideration—a critical part, in fact, to our disruptive solution to the epidemic of chronic pain. This annual membership model works for the company and works for most of our clients. In fact, I would argue that it aids our outcomes.

Radiant clients are investing in themselves as much as they're investing in us.

Our clients are choosing to spend the money—sometimes making sacrifices to do so because they genuinely want to get better. This improves the psychology of the therapy and makes the patient a committed partner with us in the process of improving their pain.

Because of this model and the ongoing nature of the therapy, with periodic boosters needed throughout the year, we develop relationships with our patients that are not typically found in other care environments. We see our clients more frequently than most other clinical environments do, and typically they're on a path of remarkable restoration. This is amazing to be a part of. Bonding and celebration are very common, and we get to know our clients in a profound and enjoyable way, in large part because this payment model facilitates this type of access.

It's not transactional. It's relational. It is almost familial.

We also use this membership concept and our model to change the experience further. Though I haven't often used the term in this book, at Radiant our patients, our clients are called "members." They are members of an exclusive club of brave, empowered, educated people. They are taking ownership and taking control back, to move towards a more fulfilling and productive life—no longer limited because of pain, and not dulled out because of some lousy drug.

Pricing is a critical piece to our model, to the viability of our business, and to the appeal we offer to our members. Indeed, we're unable to serve everyone, but we've made it affordable to most, as well as being as flexible as possible to an appropriate level. Undoubtedly, some will argue that without insurance coverage it is not sustainable, but I fully and completely disagree. To some, insurance coverage does offer a stamp of validity, but in my mind, that is a stamp of validity from the institution we're seeking to disrupt. Our members want a better experience and a better outcome, and they're willing to invest in that—to invest in us and to invest in themselves. We have years of experience and hundreds of people who have seen value in our solution and pricing, and I am confident that will increase substantially as we grow.

PLACE

A Radiant Pain Relief Centres' treatment room is set up for only one purpose: to create the best experience possible for our clients. Our treatment rooms are comfortable, even spa-like. The exam table found in most medical clinics is replaced with a very comfortable recliner chair. Pillows, blankets, water, tea, music, and soothing colors and lights are all part of the Radiant Pain Relief Centres experience, and these things are not typically found in any clinical setting, from hospitals to private practices. In our minds, the patient experience is critical to the outcome and the value of the investment they are making in our therapy.

A Radiant Pain Relief Centre is a space of about 1500 square feet. It has four treatment rooms, with four devices able to operate simultaneously. This creates maximum efficiency, allowing us to serve the greatest number of people in the most efficient way. We have a dedicated space for all new client presentations, which is quiet and inviting, and of course, the necessary administrative and work space for our team. The space and the efficiency it creates are necessary for two important reasons. The first is cost containment, and the second is efficiency with maximum client experience, both of which are necessary to ensure that we can offer our therapy at an affordable price, create a phenomenal client experience, and still be profitable as a company. This is space and resource allocation not available in most clinical environments, yet one that is necessary to create a profitable operation and optimal client experience.

PROMOTION

"Promotion" is another word for advertising—how we get the word out and create an appealing invitation to take action. Without advertising, the technology would never catch the attention of the consumer world to any high degree. Look how advertising has impacted healthcare today, with pharmaceutical companies advertising to consumers and informing them to the point that they go and "request" certain medications from their physicians. No doubt, being a direct-to-consumer business is the most direct way to inform and persuade.

We have had many clients ask us, "Why haven't I heard of this before?" or "Why doesn't my doctor know about this?" Clearly, getting the message to those who hurt and whom we can help is highly important, to reach more people and to help the business. Direct-to-consumer advertising is the most effective way to get word out, particularly with the use of social media and earned media (PR, news coverage). In the early days of Radiant, we lacked a budget to do much advertising, and what we did, we did rather unsophisticatedly, yet it worked. People came. As we grow and gain the capacity and budget to advertise more, we'll push forward in a significant fashion. In these first years, as we have had limited resources and limited capacity, we have learned a few things that will go with us as we grow.

The first is story: our client stories are amazing and moving. The stories are the most compelling indication of the unique value that we can offer. The second is people: we have and intend to continue to only use actual clients in our advertising, on our website, and in all of our materials. No stock photos, just real, happy clients whose lives were previously diminished because of pain, restored back to a more normalized perception of pain. The third is education: we are not a pain clinic; we are changing the way chronic pain is understood and treated. To do this, we must lead with education. This book is part of that.

When we first started doing some digital advertising,

paying for key search words, we could get our ads to rise to the top by simply spending money. Thinking we were making it easy for them, we had a "click to call feature," meaning that from their phone with one click, a potential consumer could reach us. Many people called, few really knew whom they were calling and what we did. They wanted a drug refill or to schedule an appointment with some doctor that wasn't associated with us. If our team did a good job of explaining who we are and how we are different, and got the potential client to come in for a free demo appointment, the person did so with little prior education.

We learned and adjusted our advertising processes to be more educational. Rather than a click to call, we started driving potential clients through an educational funnel. The click took them to a video explaining our process while also giving them access to information and education about what we do. Even the process of securing a free demo is one that reinforces the learning by asking clients certain questions about their pain, but also about their "why": why now, why they and their families need them out of pain now. Through that education funnel, the clients come to us, primed, educated, thinking about why they want to get out of pain, and feeling differently about their engagement with us.

Our therapy is about changing lives, and our promotional efforts are designed to reflect that.

PEOPLE

While not traditionally considered one of the Ps of Marketing, "people" is sometimes added as a consideration. In a high-touch, interpersonal, highly individual process like our therapy, the people aspect of how we think is critical. The technology we use is incredible. But without capable hands to operate it and, more importantly, caring hearts to connect with our clients, it is a static instrument. I already talked about the mantra "the best technology, the best people, the best experience," with the people being the key to bridging the technology to an experience, but I want to share a bit more about how we think about our team.

We look at our business as having a tremendous opportunity and a tremendous responsibility. Disrupting such a significant industry and building such a different approach to such a significant problem requires passion, hard work, execution, intelligence, bravery, compassion, patience, and more. We require a lot of our employees, but we work hard to empower them with knowledge and skill development, not just technically or scientifically, but personally. We invest in putting all of our team in courses and training, such as Brendon Burchard's High Performance Academy, to help them develop from within the mindset, confidence, and habits that will help them perform at their best. We have intentionally integrated personal development into our training process and into our culture. We believe that high-performing companies start with high-performing people.

MODEL FOR DISRUPTION

I hope that this chapter provided some valuable insights into how we've thought differently about building Radiant. The business aspect of what we do is important. We feel that being able to think about these aspects and build them with the mindset of what would be optimal versus making them fit within the confines of an existing business structure, such as a clinic or hospital, has allowed us to build an equally important complement to our therapy. Both have to be present for success. In addition to the thinking that has framed the development of our business, we have worked hard to create a culture that is focused on continuous improvement, development, and growth that will allow us to continually deliver value to our clients at a higher and higher level.

CHAPTER 6

THE CHALLENGE OF CHALLENGING THE STATUS QUO

———

The secret of change is to focus all of your energy, not on fighting the old, but on building the new.

—SOCRATES

This chapter discusses business challenges, and the resistance and struggle faced in building and gaining traction for Radiant.

It's probably very appropriate that a disruptive solution to chronic pain would be very difficult to get off the ground because chronic pain itself is so difficult, complicated, and nuanced. In some ways, anything other than a challenging journey would not do justice to the difficulty and complexity of a life in pain. The story and process of building Radiant, as I'll share throughout this chapter, is one of challenge, perseverance, and never giving up—much like the stories of patients who must choose to keep going in the face of difficult, painful conditions. At the end of the day, we can't always control our circumstances, but we can control how we respond to them. I hope that, as I share this part of the Radiant story and my own personal trials, it will help to inform how all of us can think about ourselves and our difficulties—whether it's a life limited because of chronic pain or something else. Struggle, pain, and disappointment are part of the human experience, and we all benefit from support, love, and compassion for others and ourselves. I am in awe of our clients who choose positivity despite the pain, and who embrace a new approach despite having been disappointed with their former therapies. I think we have the best clients in the world because of this—they are their own band of believers and achievers.

MY PERSONAL STORY OF STRUGGLE

Prior to starting Radiant, I played key operations and business development roles with two young companies that became growth award winners and made their owners rich. It is a lot of fun working in a young company that is growing. The energy is infectious, and I loved it and knew that someday I wanted to be in the driver's seat of such a company. By day I lived a productive, busy, and engaging life. I was liked; I was important and valued. Work was fun and energetically rewarding. However, my personal life was a mess.

My wife and I had moved our young family from the Phoenix area to the Portland, Oregon, area in the summer of 2006. In Arizona, we had just built a new home and put most of our money into it. When we decided to move our family to Portland—to raise our three young kids, ages five, three, and one at the time, in a cooler and greener place (literally and figuratively)—the real estate market in Arizona was still going strong. We didn't expect to find the challenges we did in selling our brand-new home. To make a long, emotional story short: thinking our home in Arizona had sold, we bought a home in Oregon, only to see the sale of the house in Arizona fall through.

This was the start of the real estate crisis which hit the country hard, and Arizona especially hard. After a few months of trying to keep both mortgages paid on a salary that could probably barely support one, we exhausted our savings. Credit card bills added up as we just tried to keep food on the table, not realizing the market was not going to get better. Inevitably, personal bankruptcy became the only way out of the debt and the burden of two devalued houses. As a provider, as a husband, and as a dad of a young family, being in this position was a personal hell for me. I felt trapped, helpless, and useless. As my wife and I faced the reality of losing everything—our home, car, credit (what was left of it)—the weight of that was overwhelming. I felt very much to blame, yet completely helpless to solve the problem myself.

In addition to this financial strain, the challenges of my wife's health were also increasing. With limited financial resources, and just as limited emotional reserves, we sought solutions across the spectrum of care to help her feel better and overcome the chronic illness she had been stoically facing for many years. Living with or being close to someone who bravely faces illness with grace and gratitude is an amazing experience. Like many of our clients, my wife became a seeker—searching out solutions and ideas that her doctors didn't have time to find, becoming her own best advocate. Most of the time I was not as supportive, patient, or understanding as she deserved, and when I think back on how she must have felt all those years—not only because of the illness, but also because of a lack of answers—I am even more awed by her bravery and strength.

Around me were people excelling, making money, living fun carefree lives, receiving accolades, and enjoying the fruits of success. Yet here I was in financial ruin, stressed, discouraged, and feeling pretty incapable of helping my wife or improving my situation. It was an interesting place to live, between these two worlds, the experience of such heavy, emotional, hard trials contrasted against success and achievement around me. It seemed for many years that it was just about survival. There was never enough money, never adequate answers for my wife's illness, never any reprieve from what felt like the crushing burdens of life. We had only one choice: to keep going, to try to choose to be positive, to try to keep trying.

Probably more than anything else, these two experiences informed and fueled my desire to build Radiant. I wanted to build something exciting. But I also wanted to do something important that would help the world by easing suffering and increasing hope. Of course I wanted to make money too, but it was more about making money to put my family in a better position, one in which I would never again have to face losing my home. Losing everything in bankruptcy just about broke me. I hated everything about it, but it was my wake-up call and it catapulted me into focusing on what really matters: my family, my relationships, and my experiences, particularly shared experiences with people I love.

So, while money was a motivating factor in building Radiant, it was more about making meaning out of my contributions to this world, protecting the people I love, and creating more opportunities for meaningful experiences for them and with them. I have felt guided and supported by something much greater than myself along the journey of creating Radiant. And although my wife didn't suffer from chronic pain, her journey paralleled the journey of those who visited our clinic. I began to understand her better; I understood our clients better. My compassion grew, as did my love for this business. Ultimately, my wife healed from chronic illness using a program based on the principles of neuroplasticity I explained in earlier chapters of this book. Her journey, our journey, has been interwoven into what Radiant is today. And this journey has been my fuel to keep pressing on even when the odds have been against me.

In retrospect, these difficult years that we lived through also built in me, and in my family, the fortitude it takes to start a company and stick with it. As a family, we were used to living on little, making sacrifices, and choosing to keep going, even when it's hard. I would need all of that fortitude and more in the next phase of the company. In many ways, I am probably not the expected person to build a business like this: not rich, not Ivy League educated, not super well-connected, and not a physician or scientist, but my life experience as much as my professional experience has thrust me into it. I saw an opportunity with the technology and a different type of model. I saw that it worked and had the potential to help a lot of people, and I felt compelled to build it. At each difficult juncture and trial,

I became more and more committed to it. Unfortunately, not everyone felt that way.

THE DAY BEFORE SOMETHING IS A SUCCESS IT IS A CRAZY IDEA

"The day before something is truly a breakthrough, it's a crazy idea. And crazy ideas are very risky to attempt" is a quote from Peter Diamandis. Peter Diamandis (Google him if you don't know that name) thinks and acts on a different level than most humans. His success as an entrepreneur is literally otherworldly; he is an inspiration to entrepreneurs and all people everywhere. In this quote is the recognition that all breakthroughs were, at some point prior, crazy ideas.

To suggest that we have a better, safer, more consistently effective and appealing solution to the epidemic of chronic pain is a crazy idea. To suggest that the approaches to chronic pain management that solely address the tissue, or are drug-based are limited, flawed, and incapable of effectively solving this problem is a crazy idea. To suggest that we can build a new business outside of the confines of traditional healthcare, without insurance and with limited physician involvement is a crazy idea. And even to suggest that I, having never built a hugely successful company, am capable of attracting the people, capital, and resources to do it is a crazy idea.

There are many reasons why this is a crazy idea. But, to quote another amazing entrepreneur, Elon Musk, "When something is important enough, you do it even if the odds are not in your favor." And so, we choose to keep moving forward because we do see it as vitally important, even when it's hard, a crazy idea, and the odds have not been in our favor.

I spent a lot of my time over the last few years defending this idea and explaining why it will work, despite it being a crazy idea. And indeed, the odds have not been in our favor. When I originally wrote this chapter, I went into great detail about this process. I realized that the level of detail and specifics about why it has been hard and how we/I chose to pivot, learn, hear (or reject) the criticism and keep going didn't really serve the purpose of this book. However, I think it is valuable to share a quick review of some of the facts to frame the uniqueness and value of what we're focused on doing.

When companies have to raise money, as we do, in order to secure and develop technology, open new centers, market, and expand influence, they do it in a few ways. They raise money privately or they go public, meaning they raise money from the general public, which requires certain disclosures, legal processes, and registrations. Historically and generally speaking, this has been a very expensive process reserved for mature, already successful companies who could afford it. We have chosen to do a RegA+. The RegA+ process is basically a legal mechanism to conduct a robust crowdfunded campaign and raise money publicly from individuals who want to own and contribute to something they see value in. It is much less costly and less burdensome, and more appropriate for younger, smaller companies like Radiant.

Without the proper legal structure, it is against the law for companies to openly solicit investment; they must only approach "accredited" investors. Without going into detail, this is essentially high net-worth individuals (angel investors), or institutional investors like seed funds, venture capital funds, and private equity groups. It is impossible to convey the full reality of the process, costs, time, emotion, energy, and more that it takes to go through the process of raising money. Experienced, highly successful people can recount many tales of the struggle of raising money, especially in the early days, especially on a "crazy idea" business. It is a brutal, humbling, challenging process.

Despite rarely having criticism for what we were doing (everyone was supportive of the idea of a better solution to the pain problem and a viable alternative to opioids), we were told "no" well over one hundred times—more if you count the investor groups who never even got back to us. Most of the time the "no" had to do with fit. We weren't a fit to their model or investment focus, or company stage, etc. The reasons for "no" were many. Here is a partial list:

You're too unproven; too early stage; too late stage; the model is not right, this has never been done before, the management team is not experienced enough; it works in "weird" Portland, but will it work in other places in the US?; sounds too good to be true; cost structure is too high, don't build clinics, just sell devices; you want to build a healthcare company that doesn't use insurance or rely upon doctors?; you don't own/didn't invent this technology; if it is so good why haven't I heard of it/why hasn't it taken off faster?; you didn't go to the right business school; you really think you can beat the pharmaceutical companies and change pain treatment away from drugs? Etc., etc., etc. On and on. No after no.

All of these criticisms are fine. There is truth in most of them, but at the end of the day, we kept moving forward, kept trying because we didn't accept the rejection. We didn't accept their version of reality; we chose to create our own. Why? Because we saw things differently. We knew all it would take was a break to move us from a crazy idea to a breakthrough. We knew the therapy worked; we knew our vision for further expansion and improvement of the therapy would only make it better. We knew the pricing structure worked and would only become more accepted with more social proof. We knew the model worked and would be more readily accepted as it grew. We just needed the capital to expand it, to grow our influence, and to louden our message.

THE PEOPLE'S SOLUTION

Of course, not everyone rejected us. In fact, it was mostly the "institutional" investors who rely upon complex financial models, historical precedent, and group thinking that said no. Until it is a success it is a crazy idea. But their success models are based upon what success has historically looked like, not innovative, disruptive solutions. Most original businesses spend a lot more time being a "crazy idea" than people realize. Overnight successes are rarely made overnight.

In time, I learned that, like the rejection I faced from traditional healthcare in trying to market this technology to them, the rejection by traditional institutional investment groups was based more in their limited thinking and constraints than a true commentary on what we were building. It began to bother me less, and I spent a lot less time and money chasing it.

The individual investor for whom chronic pain is a relevant problem, and who perhaps has been impacted personally or has had family impacted, was our biggest champion. Most of those we met with, who could, did invest. Just as with our clients, it was the individual that has been the early adopter, investing with us because they like the mission as much as the potential upside. The challenge was that this is a very slow, manual process, transacting the money raised person by person, individual investment by individual investment. It is very hard to raise a lot of money quickly in this way, an individual transaction at a time. This is one of the main reasons we have been drawn to the RegA+ path, as it allows us to leverage more people who have an aligned interest and values more quickly and on a larger scale.

Of course, this decision brought with it criticism from some—particularly those from an institutional capital background—about it being risky, the wrong approach, and the less sustainable approach. But at the end of the day, Radiant's success lies in the client, the average person that we help, so I feel that it is totally appropriate that its financial success is tied to the same group of people. Nothing would make me happier than to see Radiant rise to change the way chronic pain is understood and treated, to change the lives of many people, and to have the company's success benefit those same people.

Radiant Pain Relief Centres is the people's solution—not the broken, antiquated, misaligned institutions of big pharma, big corporation, traditional thinking healthcare and industry. It is progressive therapy for progressive thinkers and early adopters, both on the treatment side and the investment side.

CHAPTER 7

THE FUTURE OF CHRONIC PAIN MANAGEMENT

―――――

The business enterprise has two—and only two—basic functions: marketing and innovation.

—PETER DRUCKER

This last chapter recaps the complex environment of pain management from a medical standpoint and lays out Radiant's vision for a better solution to the epidemic of chronic pain.

If you or someone you care about is dealing with chronic pain, if that pain is interfering with life, and if the current treatment options that have been tried are not working, or the side effects too significant of a concern, there is great news. The future of chronic pain treatment is here. It is safe. It is consistently effective for nearly all types of chronic pain. And it is much more appealing than what has been offered before. In this last chapter, I will outline the Radiant Pain Relief Centres model and vision for changing the way chronic pain is treated. Before I do, I just want to recap the factors that necessitate this model being the optimal way to combine the latest pain science, innovation therapies, and enhanced client experience to change the way chronic pain is understood and treated.

THE PAIN PROBLEM AND THE RADIANT SOLUTION

Chronic pain is a huge problem. It is a complicated problem which most clinical professionals touch in some way. Yet most of the therapies that exist are limited, outdated, and inconsistent approaches that address the tissue only or are a drug with impact to the entire chemistry of the body. For these reasons, the current treatment options are often ineffective, and may in fact be risky, dangerous, or addictive.

The science now clearly indicates that chronic pain becomes a problem of the brain—all pain comes from the brain, but in chronic pain the brain becomes fixated on the pain. It becomes "wired" to expect the pain, to cause the pain to grow, to perceive it as the new normal rather than a temporary indicator of a problem in which the pain is serving a protective and productive purpose.

Despite the lack of consistently effective therapies for chronic pain, there is an economic disincentive to innovate and disrupt from within the industry. For this reason, we're building a new approach.

Like other companies that have disrupted their industries with new technology, new models, and new thinking, (e.g. Uber, Airbnb, Tesla), Radiant Pain Relief Centres is changing the way chronic pain is understood and treated, and is delivering a better therapy through a better model, directly to the consumer—choosing to innovate and to think outside of the confines of traditional, institutional healthcare business operations and economics.

Instead, the focus is on the consumer, the pain sufferer. They are the master that is served, and that switch has allowed an economic alignment to unfold throughout the supply chain from consumer, to care delivery, to supplier/manufacturer, to investor/shareholder. But Radiant, much like in the other notable disrupters, starts with the end user, and creating, offering, and delivering value there first. This value then translates to revenues, profits, and shareholder value. Earlier chapters of this book discuss the economics of the Radiant Pain Relief Centres model, so I won't reiterate those here, except to say a key aspect of our business thesis and model is affordability and value for the consumer. The rest, we believe, will take care of itself as we focus on growth and sensible stewardship of the operations.

The Radiant model is a client model—a consumer-facing and consumer-focused model. It's a consumer business that just happens to be addressing a healthcare problem. Like any successful business or brand, it is built upon delivering value, consistently different from or superior to what the competition is offering. Like other disruptive businesses, it is built around thinking and delivering differently than others have done before. For Radiant, it starts with the therapy but extends far beyond that.

Rather than just masking the pain with a drug, an injection, or some physical approach to the tissue, Radiant is pioneering and developing therapies that go to the root of chronic pain, which is the brain. Our therapies safely and effectively retrain the brain, restoring it back to a more normalized perception of pain. The result is consistent, significant, often total relief that becomes lasting for nearly all types of chronic pain, without the side effects and risks of the other therapies that have existed previously. The therapy is different, novel, better, and disruptive, but the economics and operating realties (client and clinical time, training, opportunity costs) of it will not work equally well within the confines of the existing medical infrastructure. A better approach requires a better delivery. In fact, this means it must be delivered outside of the world of traditional medical infrastructure.

A DIFFERENT APPROACH, A DIFFERENT RESULT

Radiant Pain Relief Centres offer a clinical environment, a care experience, and a pricing structure that is unmatched anywhere in healthcare.

Unlike most medical/clinical environments that are cold and sterile, Radiant Pain Relief Centres are warm, inviting, and spa-like. They are accessible and patient-centric. Because this therapy is the exclusive focus of care at Radiant Pain Relief Centres, we have developed a level of expertise and acumen that can never be replicated by anyone who does it part time, or who dabbles in it in conjunction with other therapies and approaches. We institutionalize the learning that inevitably comes from volume and experience. This allows us to create a level of consistency to deliver care, and to offer an experience that cannot be found elsewhere. This consistency and the improved client experience are necessary to build a strong brand, to build a disruptive brand. They work together: therapy and experience. Both are necessary components of real disruption, of real change, and of delivering a superior solution.

Our model couples innovative therapy with improved

client experience to create a better result. Through systems and processes, we create a level of clinical and operating consistency that allows for us to build a strong, disruptive brand and shift thinking around this monumental problem. We have made this cutting-edge therapy affordable though a pricing model that simultaneously promotes optimal usage, driving better outcomes and profitable operations.

INVESTING IN A FULL LIFE

Even though there is a cost, most patients tell us that it's the best investment they've made in the management of their pain. Our clients are choosing to spend the money—sometimes making sacrifices to do so because they genuinely want to get better. This improves the psychology of the therapy and makes the patient a committed partner with us in the process of improving their pain.

Because of this model and the ongoing nature of the therapy, with periodic boosters needed throughout the year, we develop relationships with our patients that are not typically found in other care environments, as we see our people more. Remember, we see our clients daily for one hour for the first few weeks as they begin on this path of remarkable and exciting restoration, which is amazing to be a part of, and then periodically, as needed, when they come in for booster treatments over the remaining months. Bonding and celebration are very common, and we get to know our clients in a profound and enjoyable way, in large part because of this payment model.

It's not transactional. It's relational. It is almost familial.

SOCIAL PROOF AND CULTURAL ADOPTION

Our client outcomes are consistently positive and dramatic. The testimonials and success stories are moving and inspiring. These are driving a social shift and building proof that is more valid and more important than any clinical study results, because it's real and personal, similar to how Starbucks proved people are willing to pay more for coffee than history and traditional thinking would have suggested, and how Apple proved that people are willing to spend hundreds on a phone, and do it every two years or so. These are two examples of social proof justifying prices for products that were either historically unprecedented or completely novel, and Radiant will do the same. In fact, the elasticity of price for reclaiming life from chronic pain safely, consistently, and effectively is certainly not like that of most other products or services.

Given the value of our offering, we could likely command a lot more, but we choose to model it, to price it in a way that is accessible to most people. It is intentional to offer our remarkable solution at a price that is reasonable. Because of the history of "snake oil" and the skepticism faced previously, I don't want anyone feeling that Radiant has taken advantage of people. I am thrilled about our pricing structure and all the benefits it accomplishes now. I am also thrilled about how our model and our pricing will evolve as we grow. Let me share some of that with you.

THIS IS THE FUTURE OF CHRONIC PAIN MANAGEMENT

This is the future of chronic pain management. It is safe. It is consistently effective. And in its totality, it is much more appealing than anything else to come before it. I believe all of that completely. And it will be more. As we grow, we will unveil three segments to our product/services suite. The first is what we have been focusing on in this book: the therapy. The second and third are education and experience, respectively. For each of these, we will be rolling out various pricing tiers based upon the value package it includes. I won't break down each of these three product/service suites and the offerings that will be included in them in great detail, but I'll explain the vision for them.

Our members come to us in chronic pain, and that pain has taken its toll on them. To some degree or another, it has minimized them, veiled their reality with this haze of discomfort—physical discomfort, but usually also emotional, mental, and spiritual discomfort. It has been said that "We don't see the world as it is, but we see it as we are." So, for a chronic pain sufferer, everything becomes filtered through this experiential lens of pain.

Like an alien virus, to some extent, the pain becomes part of them, part of their identity. It limits the activities they can do. Recreational activities, work activities, and normal daily life activities all become harder, shorter, or are lost altogether. This eats the bandwidth of cognitive functioning. Chronic pain is discouraging, it's hard, it's isolating, and for some it's even dehumanizing. But as people are treated at Radiant and as they find an effective resolution to their pain, some, most, and even ultimately all, of their activities, their work, their normal life, and their humanness can be reclaimed. It happens quickly. The initial consultation and demo is the start, and for most of our members it is a process of weeks, not years, to reclaim substantial ground that has been lost in all of these areas.

To be able to resolve their pain without complicating them further because of some drug side effect that disrupts sleep or mental acuity, allows them to become less complicated. They need fewer drugs to function. They feel better. They sleep better. They move better. They think clearer. Hope is restored. Life is restored. And as this onion layer is peeled away, as the veil of pain is lifted, they start to see themselves as fully human again. Many of our members lose weight, and improve their relationships and their productive outputs in work, hobbies, and life, simply because they're getting better and becoming less complicated in terms of their health.

These transformations from a restricted life because of pain back to a regular life where pain isn't the daily disruptor anymore are astonishing, life-changing, and life-saving for many people. It happens naturally, but Radiant will help it happen with greater intention by creating various offerings that expand the education to include neuroscience, neuroplasticity, exercise physiology, nutrition, and even personal development. We are creating programs to expand how each patient can experience life, celebrate life, and thrive in life. We call these programs and aspects of our business "Radiant Life" and "Radiant Learning," respectively. This focus on education and experience, as well as therapy, will work collectively to create a Radiant Life for all of our members that choose to pursue it.

AN INVITATION TO JOIN WITH US

Radiant Pain Relief Centres are the future of chronic pain management. ST is a safer, more effective, more appealing therapy for all of us who have been touched by this epidemic. We are expanding and empowering education about chronic pain and helping people move beyond a life of pain. We are growing through corporate-owned centers, through strategic partnerships with other clinical/healthcare professionals, and through franchises, all operating under our brand, clinical protocol, business systems, and Positive Experience Process (PEP). Our vision is to grow this therapy, to shift understanding about chronic pain, and to build the safest, most consistently effective treatment for it.

Our approach doesn't just mask the pain or numb people out, it enables more people to thrive in their world, in the world we all share. Radiant Pain Relief Centers offer a superior patient experience with a graduating path of tools and resources to experience life to its fullest. This is the future of chronic pain management. It doesn't stop with treating the pain. It uses the resolution of pain and the education about the brain as a springboard to more. This is a social enterprise, changing lives and communities. This is progressive healthcare, delivering superior care in an artful, thoughtful, graceful, and consistent way. This is disruptive business, stepping outside of the norm, thinking differently, acting differently, and delivering differently. And this is uniquely Radiant.

It is my hope that as you've read this, you've seen it as I see it, as we at Radiant see it, and that you will join with us, as a member, a referrer, an advocate, an investor—some type of participant in our efforts to change the world by changing the way chronic pain is understood and treated.

Thank you,
Brendon

ABOUT THE AUTHORS

———

P. BRENDON LUNDBERG is a previous chronic pain sufferer with deep experience in healthcare management, marketing, business development, and sales. He played key operational and business development roles for two award-winning companies and was director of sales and marketing for a medical start-up. Brendon lives with his wife and children near Portland, Oregon.

DAVID B. FARLEY, MD, is the chief medical officer of Radiant Pain Relief Centres and has treated patients for thirty years in his family practice. Dr. Farley earned his medical degree from the joint Harvard–MIT Program of Health Sciences and Technology. He and his wife live in West Linn, Oregon.

Made in the USA
San Bernardino, CA
07 August 2018